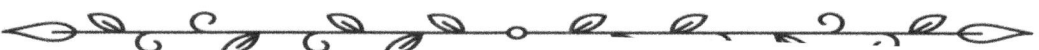

HERBAL ANTIBIOTICS

Over 150 Natural Remedies for Overcoming Any Ailment.

*A Reliable Access to Nature's Healing Wonders
in the Age of Antibiotic Resistance*

Flora Fernhart

Unlock a World of Books Before Anyone Else!

WE INVITE YOU TO JOIN OUR ELITE READERS' INNER CIRCLE!

As an elite reader, you will have the unique opportunity to access our preview books <u>for free</u>

(e.g. you could have read this book, in preview, for free)

SCAN THE QR CODE OR VISIT

<u>wiseapublishing.com/innercircle/join</u>

Receive a <u>Complimentary Book</u> from Our Entire Collection as Your <u>Welcome Gift</u>

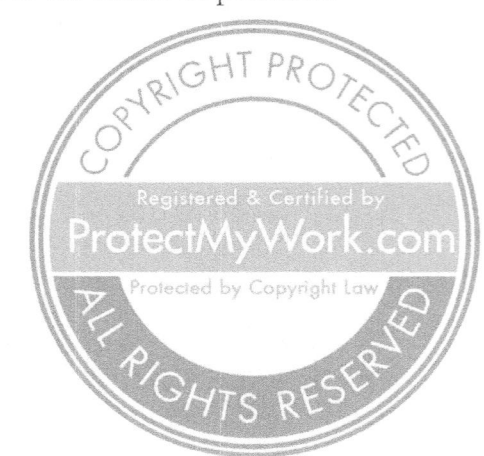

Table of contents

ENJOY YOUR EXCLUSIVE BONUSES! 5

INTRODUCTION 6

HERBAL ANTIBIOTICS REVOLUTION: WHY IT MATTERS 8
The Rise of Antibiotic Resistance 9
The Limitations of Traditional Antibiotics 10
The Power of Herbal Antibiotics 10
The Science Behind Herbal Antibiotics 11
The Role of Herbal Antibiotics 12
The Future of Herbal Antibiotics 13
Summary 14

UNDERSTANDING ANTIBIOTIC RESISTANCE: A BRIEF OVERVIEW 15
Antibiotic Resistance: Definition 15
The Mechanism of Antibiotic Resistance 17
The Causes of Antibiotic Resistance 19
Herbal Antibiotics as Alternate Medication 20
The Impact of Antibiotic Resistance 21
Combating Antibiotic Resistance 23
Summary 24

POWER OF NATURE: AN INTRODUCTION TO HERBAL ANTIBIOTICS 25
History of Herbal Antibiotics 26
How did Pharmacology come into being? 27
How Herbal Antibiotics Work? 27
The Benefits of Herbal Antibiotics 29
Common Misconceptions about Herbal Antibiotics 30
Summary 31

SUSTAINABLE AND ETHICAL HERB GATHERING 32
The Importance of Sustainability in Herb Gathering 32
Understanding Ethical Herb Gathering 33
Principles of Sustainable and Ethical Herb Gathering 34
Practical Tips for Sustainable and Ethical Herb Gathering 36
The Role of Community in Sustainable Herb Gathering 37
Summary 38

GROWING YOUR OWN HERB GARDEN: A STEP-BY-STEP GUIDE 39
The Benefits of Growing Your Own Home Garden 39
Choosing the Right Herbs for Your Garden 40
Planning Your Herbal Garden 41
Planting and Caring for Your Herbs: A Step-by-Step Process 42
Harvesting and Storing Herbs 44
Summary 46

TOP HERBAL ANTIBIOTICS: DETAILED PROFILES AND USES 47
Introduction to Herbal Profiles 47

Types of Herbal Antibiotics 47

Echinacea 48

Garlic 50

Ginger 52

Goldenseal 54

Oregano 56

Thyme 58

Turmeric 60

Summary 62

PRACTICAL APPLICATIONS: HERBAL ANTIBIOTICS FOR COMMON AILMENTS 63

Introduction to Practical Applications 63

Common Cold and Flu 64

Urinary Tract Infections 65

Skin Infections 66

Respiratory Infections 67

Digestive Issues 69

Preventive Measures and Boosting Immunity 70

Summary 71

RECIPES FOR HEALTH: MAKING YOUR OWN HERBAL ANTIBIOTICS 72

Echinacea Tincture for Immune Support 73

Garlic Oil for Ear Infections 74

Ginger Tea for Digestive Health 75

Goldenseal Salve for Skin Infection 76

Oregano Capsules for Respiratory Health 77

Thyme Syrup for Cough 78

Turmeric Paste for Inflammation 79

More Natural Remedies 80

Summary 80

THE FUTURE OF HERBAL ANTIBIOTICS: TRENDS AND PREDICTIONS 81

Current Trends in Herbal Antibiotics 81

Emerging Research in Herbal Antibiotics 82

Predictions for Future Herbal Antibiotics 83

Role of Herbal Antibiotics in Global Health 85

Preparing for the Future: How to Stay Informed 86

Summary 88

CONCLUSION: 89

YOUR JOURNEY TOWARDS NATURAL HEALTH 89

Enjoy your exclusive bonuses!

Dear Reader,

As a token of our appreciation for joining us on this enlightening journey into herbal healing, we are thrilled to offer you **3 exclusive bonuses** designed to enrich your experience and deepen your understanding of natural remedies. These special resources have been carefully selected to complement the knowledge you've gained from our book and to further empower you in your exploration of herbalism.

To access these invaluable resources, simply click on the link below

www.wiseapublishing.com/herbalAB/bonus/
or scan the QR code.

Here's a glimpse into the bonuses that await you:

Free Video Course on Herbalism for Beginners: Dive deeper into the world of herbal medicine with our comprehensive video course. Designed specifically for beginners, this course offers a dynamic and engaging way to learn about the power and potential of herbal remedies.

Exclusive Access to Our Herbalist Community: Become part of a vibrant and supportive community of like-minded individuals who share your passion for herbalism. Whether you're seeking advice, looking to share your own discoveries, or simply wanting to engage with others on your herbal journey, our community is here to welcome you with open arms.

Bonus Book on Crystals and Stones: Expand your knowledge of natural healing with our special bonus book dedicated to the use of crystals and stones for wellness. This comprehensive guide explores the unique properties and uses of various crystals and stones, offering practical advice on how to incorporate them into your healing practices.

We hope these bonuses will enhance your journey into herbal healing and provide you with additional tools and knowledge to explore the fascinating world of natural remedies.

Thank you for choosing to embark on this journey with us.

Introduction

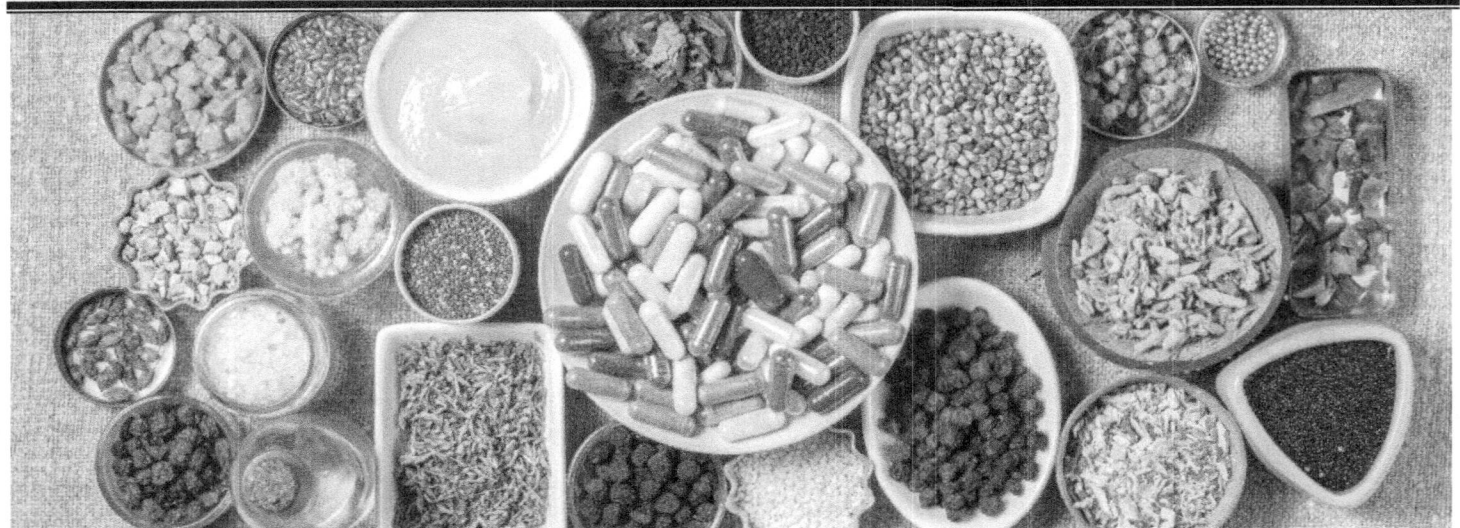

From the era of natural healing with herbs and plants that were easily available in the surroundings of our ancestors, we have waived off the path of natural healing for way too long now. Antibiotics and other drugs have taken over the market but also our bodies.

There are always increasing concerns over antibiotic resistance and adverse side effects of synthetic drugs; the quest for safer and more effective alternatives has led many to explore the world of herbal antibiotics. Herbal antibiotics are natural remedies derived from plants that possess antimicrobial properties.

Herbal Antibiotics, also known as phyto-chemicals, refer to natural compounds found in plants with antimicrobial properties, which means they can help fight off harmful microorganisms such as bacteria, viruses, fungi, and parasites. They're an integral part of plant immunity, but humans have also used them for centuries as natural remedies for various health issues.

Various cultures have owned these ancient remedies, dating to the Stone Age; solutions and medications are available to combat infections and promote healing without the harmful effects often associated with conventional antibiotics.

In this journey through the realm of herbal antibiotics, we will explore their history, efficacy, and safety as a viable passage to natural healing. Let us embark on a voyage to discover the treasures nature has bestowed upon us in the form of these potent botanical healers that are still unavailable for us to reach out to.

Civilizations such as ancient Egypt, China, and India have a rich history of herbal antibiotics. Herbal antibiotics have been vital in treating infections, injuries, and diseases long before the advent of synthetic drugs. The knowledge passed down through generations has paved the way for modern research to delve deeper into the healing potential of these plant-based medicines.

The herbs, plants, and other nature-gifted treasures are rich in natural compounds. These natural compounds, such as alkaloids, flavonoid, and essential oils, have shown the ability to target and inhibit the growth of harmful bacteria, viruses, and fungi. Unlike conventional antibiotics that target a specific bacterial strain, herbal antibiotics may have broader antimicrobial properties, offering a holistic approach to combating infections.

One of the primary advantages of herbal antibiotics is their potential to mitigate antibiotic resistance. As these remedies often utilize multiple active compounds, bacteria may find it harder to develop resistance than single-target synthetic drugs. Additionally, herbal antibiotics are known for their milder impact on the body, reducing the risk of adverse side effects commonly associated with conventional antibiotics. However, it is essential to strike a balance between traditional knowledge and evidence-based research to ensure their safe and effective use.

While herbal antibiotics offer promising benefits, it is crucial to acknowledge that not all herbal remedies are safe for everyone. Like any medication, these natural remedies can interact with other drugs or cause allergic reactions in some individuals. Therefore, consulting a qualified healthcare professional before incorporating herbal antibiotics into one's health regimen is essential to ensure safety and efficacy.

Herbal antibiotics present an exciting pathway to harness the healing power of nature and combat infections in a safer, more sustainable manner. With a rich history of use and growing evidence of their effectiveness, these botanical wonders offer a potential safe passage toward natural healing. As we progress through this exploration, it becomes evident that the synergy between traditional wisdom and modern science may hold the key to unlocking the full potential of herbal antibiotics in our pursuit of well-being.

Unlike synthetic antibiotics, typically designed to target one specific type of bacteria, herbal antibiotics can work against many harmful microorganisms. They also function differently, often supporting the body's natural defenses rather than directly killing pathogens.

Despite the beneficial properties of these herbal antibiotics, they should not be used as a replacement for conventional medical treatments, especially in the case of serious or persistent infections. Furthermore, it's crucial to consult with a healthcare provider before beginning any herbal regimen, as certain herbs can interact with medications or may not be safe for individuals with specific health conditions.

Over-reliance on herbal and synthetic antibiotics can contribute to antibiotic resistance, a growing global health concern.

Remember that while herbal antibiotics can be a part of a holistic health approach, they are not a magic bullet and should be used responsibly and as part of a balanced lifestyle that includes a healthy diet, regular exercise, and routine medical checkups. In some places, using conventional antibiotics is inevitable, and rightly so. No medication should be neglected, and all medication should be taken only after discussing it with your medical practitioner.

Herbal Antibiotics Revolution: Why It Matters

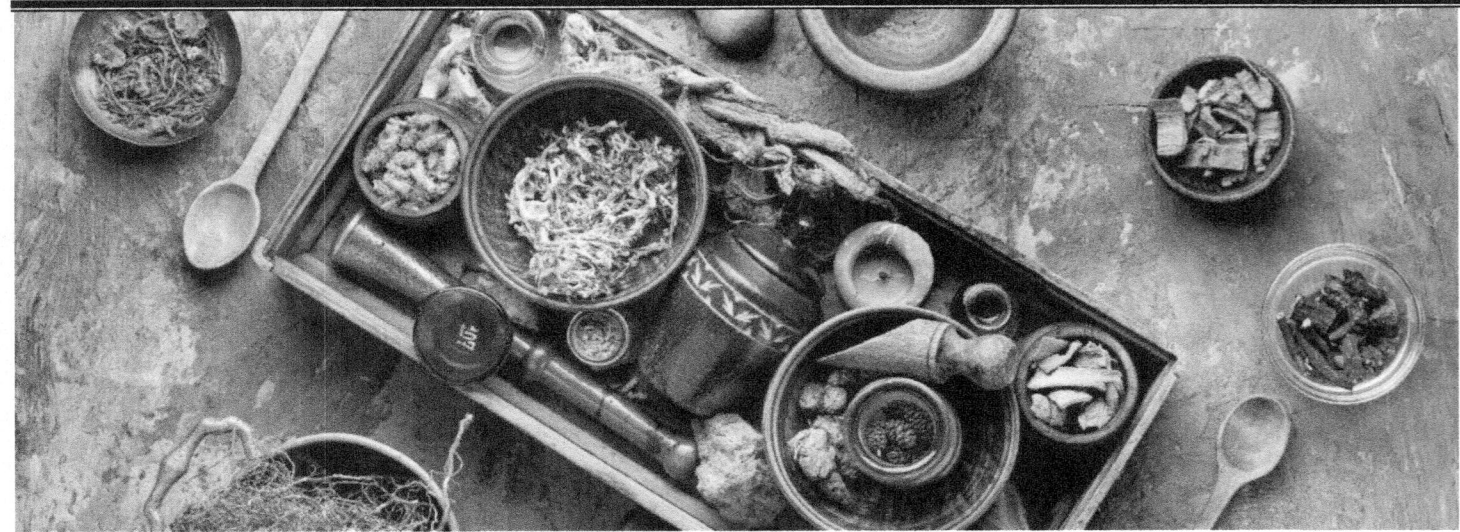

The term "herbal antibiotics revolution" describes the rising popularity and use of herbal medicines to complement prescription antibiotics. With time, it has been seen that herbal antibiotics have been in demand globally and undoubtedly consist of countless healing benefits. Natural compounds derived from plants, known as herbal antibiotics, are thought to have antibacterial characteristics and can treat various bacterial, viral, and fungal illnesses.

Several things are fueling the herbal antibiotics revolution. First, the abuse of traditional antibiotics, which has sparked the emergence of antibiotic-resistant bacteria, is a rising concern. Due to this, alternatives that efficiently cure illnesses without fostering antibiotic resistance are now required.

Secondly, a growing number of people are drawn to natural and comprehensive approaches to healthcare. Traditional medical practices like Ayurveda and Traditional Chinese Medicine have been using herbal medicines for centuries, and they are viewed as a milder and more long-lasting alternative to modern antibiotics.

The growing body of research and scientific evidence demonstrating the efficacy of some herbal medicines in treating infections is another element fueling the revolution in herbal antibiotics.

Although herbal antibiotics have gained attention and may have advantages, it's crucial to remember that they can't always replace prescription antibiotics and cannot treat severe diseases and infections. No one can deny the significance of the herbal antibiotic revolution.

The Rise of Antibiotic Resistance

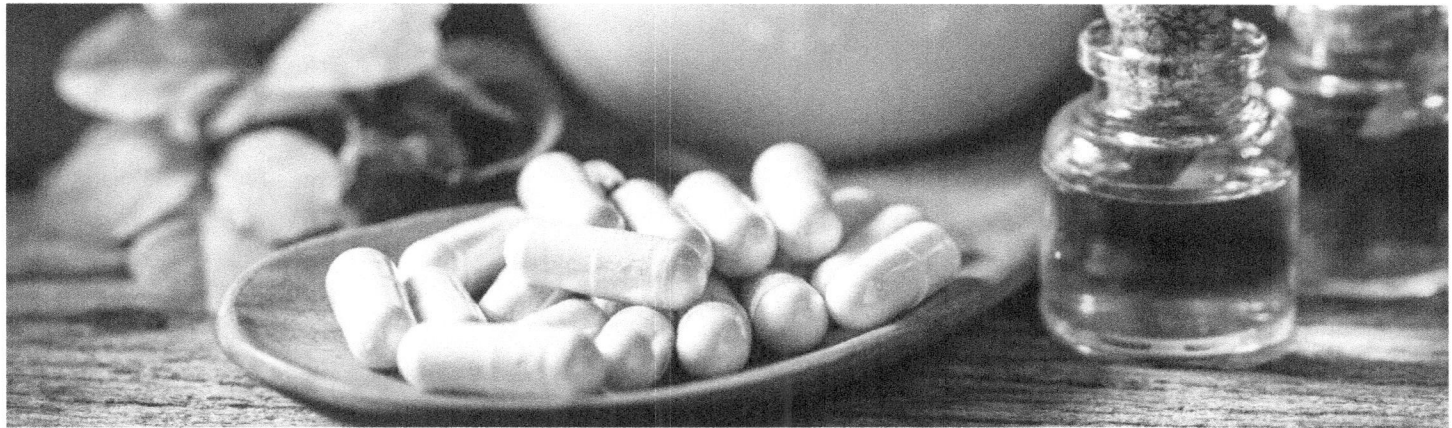

A major issue in healthcare is the emergence of antibiotic resistance. Antibiotic resistance happens when bacteria create defenses against the drugs' effects, making them useless for treating infections.

Several variables cause the rise in antibiotic resistance. Out of these, antibiotic abuse and overuse is a significant contributing factor. This involves providing medicine inappropriately, such as antibiotics for viral infections that don't respond to them. The availability of antibiotics over the counter and less knowledge of proper usage in some nations without the right regulations have also contributed to overuse.

Another significant cause is the ineffective infection control procedures in healthcare settings. The spread of resistant germs in hospitals can be facilitated by poor hand hygiene, inadequate sterilization of medical equipment, and inappropriate antibiotic use.

A further factor in the emergence of antibiotic resistance is the use of antibiotics in agriculture, particularly in animal production. In livestock, antibiotics are frequently used to enhance growth and prevent illnesses. The development of resistant microorganisms that can spread to humans through the food chain is facilitated by this pervasive use.

Antibiotic resistance has far-reaching repercussions. As infections become more difficult to treat, they increase morbidity and mortality rates. Countless factors result in antibiotic resistance; unfortunately, they are on the rise globally.

Due to extended hospital stays, the requirement for more extensive treatment choices, and the creation of new antibiotics also raise healthcare expenditures. Additionally, surgeries, cancer therapies, and other medical operations that depend on efficient infection control are at risk from antibiotic resistance.

Various tactics and remedies have been used to combat the growth in antibiotic resistance. These include enhancing antibiotic stewardship, which entails more sensible prescription techniques, instructing medical personnel and the public on the proper use of antibiotics, and implementing infection control protocols in healthcare facilities. The development of fresh antibiotics and complementary therapies is also necessary.

A serious risk to global health is occurring from the emergence of antibiotic resistance. Antibiotic resistance affects people of all age groups, so there is no definitive answer to restraining it without making the patient more ill. To ensure the right use of antibiotics and encourage the development of novel treatment options, a concerted effort from healthcare professionals, legislators, and the public is needed to address this complicated issue. However, we can't deny the fact that herbal antibiotics consist of the risk of resistance, and to control it, there are a handful of tactics only.

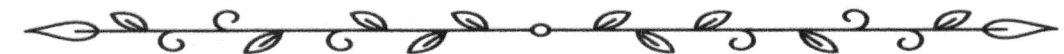

The Limitations of Traditional Antibiotics

Pharmaceutical antibiotics have been known to be dangerous if used in the wrong manner. Antibiotics can have adverse effects on health as they present with the following limitations.

1. Antibiotic Resistance:

The misuse of pharmaceutical antibiotics has led to the development of antibiotic-resistant bacteria. This is a major global health concern, making treating common infections more difficult.

2. Effect on Micro-biome:

These antibiotics do not discriminate between harmful and beneficial bacteria, often killing helpful bacteria in the gut. This can lead to an imbalance in the micro-biome, affecting digestive health and potentially leading to other health problems.

3. Cost:

Pharmaceutical antibiotics can be expensive, particularly newer or specialized ones, which might be out of reach for people in low-income areas. Even developing an antibiotic is costly for the pharmacy industry.

4. Environmental Impact:

The production and disposal of pharmaceutical antibiotics contribute to pollution, affecting water quality and soil health. This is the opposite of herbal antibiotics. Herbal antibiotics are compounds extracted from plants.

The Power of Herbal Antibiotics

Herbal medicines are a hidden weapon, ready to be released in a world where antibiotic resistance is rising, and conventional antibiotics are encountering restrictions. These plant-based natural powerhouses present a viable option in the struggle against infections. Herbal antibiotics have the potential to completely change how we treat microbial diseases due to their wide range of activity, potential synergy with conventional antibiotics, and lack of side effects.

Following are some of the potential benefits of herbal antibiotics, which also make them a strong alternative to traditional antibiotics:

- **A wider spectrum of activity:** Compared to conventional antibiotics, many herbal antibiotics are more effective against a variety of bacteria, as well as some viruses and fungi. This adaptability is useful in treating infections brought on by many pathogens.
- **Lessening the danger of antibiotic resistance:** Herbal antibiotics function in various ways, including destroying biofilms, affecting bacterial cell walls, or preventing bacterial enzymes. It is less likely for bacteria to acquire resistance to herbal medicines since these processes frequently differ from those targeted by conventional antibiotics.
- **Less adverse effects:** Compared to conventional antibiotics, herbal medicines are generally safe and can cause fewer negative effects. They have a long history of usage in conventional medical procedures and are made from natural sources. However, because they still have the potential to have negative responses or interactions, it is crucial to use them under the right supervision and with prudence.
- **Effects of synergism:** Some herbal antibiotics may enhance the efficacy of conventional antibiotics when used together. This combined therapy has the potential to shorten the course of treatment and have a stronger antibacterial effect.

- **Gut micro-biome preservation:** Unlike conventional antibiotics, which can upset the equilibrium of the gut micro-biome, some herbal antibiotics have been discovered to affect dangerous bacteria while protecting good bacteria selectively. This can lessen the chance of issues brought on by micro-biome change and preserve a healthy gut environment.

Natural antibiotics are widely accessible and reasonably priced, especially in areas with limited access to conventional treatment. They, therefore, represent a viable alternative for people who do not have access to or cannot afford conventional antibiotics.

Herbal antibiotics should not be used in place of conventional antibiotics in cases of serious or life-threatening infections, and it is crucial to remember this. Depending on the herbal cure, the concentration of the active ingredients, and individual characteristics, they could not be as effective or dependable in specific circumstances. Before utilizing herbal antibiotics, speaking with a doctor or herbalist is essential.

The Science Behind Herbal Antibiotics

Studying plant components with antibacterial activity is the basis of the science behind herbal antibiotics. For generations, people have utilized these herbal treatments to cure illnesses and infections. Recent studies have demonstrated the ability of substances like allicin in garlic, carvacrol in oregano, and berberine in golden-seal, among others, to alter the structure of bacterial cells and restrict their growth. Investigating natural medicines' potential as synthetic antibiotic alternatives requires a thorough understanding of the science behind herbal antibiotics and their efficiency.

Throughout history, societies from all over the world have employed herbal antibiotics to treat a variety of infections and illnesses. Due to the rising worry over antibiotic resistance and the negative side effects of synthetic antibiotics, interest in these natural therapies has recently increased. Research is still being done to completely understand the processes by which herbal antibiotics function, but evidence points to their potential for success in battling dangerous germs.

Garlic (Allium sativum) is one of the most well-known natural antibiotics. Allicin, a substance found in garlic, has been demonstrated to have potent antibacterial activities. By compromising the strength of bacterial cell walls, allicin promotes bacterial cell death and inhibits bacterial growth. Studies have shown that garlic extract is efficient against common germs, including Escherichia coli and Staphylococcus aureus. For instance, a study discovered that using garlic extract dramatically slowed the growth of these bacteria in lab tests. This study was published in the Journal of Antimicrobial Chemotherapy.

Oregano (Origanum vulgare), a common natural antibiotic, is another. Carvacrol, a substance found in oregano, has strong antibacterial effects. Carvacrol has been found to weaken the structure of bacterial cell membranes, allowing intra-cellular components to flow out and ultimately killing the bacterium. A study published in Microbial Ecology in Health and Disease revealed the efficiency of oregano essential oil against different bacterial strains, including ones resistant to antibiotics.

Numerous more herbs and plants have also proven to possess antibacterial characteristics in addition to these few examples. These include, among other things, tea tree oil, ginger, turmeric, and thyme. Although each herbal antibiotic may have a different mode of action, their overall efficiency and effectiveness can be related to their capacity to interfere with bacterial cell structure and metabolic processes.

Notably, herbal medicines shouldn't be used instead of prescription antibiotics for serious or life-threatening infections. Minor to severe infections can serve as an alternate treatment option or a supplement to standard medical

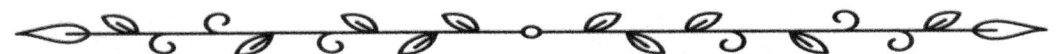

care. Additionally, using herbal antibiotics may lessen the need for synthetic antibiotics, thereby slowing the emergence of resistant germs.

Herbs are also an alternate for many basic needs of the human body. Rosemary is entering the hair care industry, and Aloe Vera is a popular plant in skin care remedies. There are numerous more.

Research has revealed that herbal antibiotics have antibacterial qualities and can be beneficial in treating bacterial illnesses. The scientific investigations that have shown their capacity to prevent the formation of hazardous germs prove their efficacy and effectiveness. Herbal medicines are a promising alternative to synthetic antibiotics and may one day help fight antibiotic-resistant bacteria. At the same time, more research is still needed to understand the science underlying their activities fully.

The Role of Herbal Antibiotics

Herbal antibiotics has a small but significant place in contemporary medicine. Herbal antibiotics are derived from natural sources, including plants, fungi, and other creatures, as opposed to conventional antibiotics, which are created from manufactured chemicals. They have been employed in conventional medical systems for many years.

Herbal antibiotics are mostly used as an alternative treatment for minor to major illnesses. They are frequently used when traditional antibiotics fail to work or have unfavorable side effects. For those who want natural therapies or have acquired antibiotic resistance, herbal antibiotics can be an alternative.

Understanding that herbal antibiotics cannot replace conventional antibiotics in cases of severe or life-threatening diseases is crucial. Since they might not be able to remove highly resistant germs completely or offer immediate relief in life-threatening conditions, their use is typically restricted to moderate infections.

The efficiency of herbal antibiotics also varies; not all claims about their efficacy have been verified by science. Speaking with medical specialists or certified naturo-paths before utilizing herbal antibiotics is essential to guarantee proper dosage and safety and rule out potential drug interactions.

The potential role of herbal antibiotics in modern medicine and their benefits for treating antibiotic-resistant infections. There is still much to learn and discover about the possible application of herbal antibiotics in contemporary medicine. Although traditional antibiotics have been used to treat bacterial infections, the growth in antibiotic resistance has sparked a greater interest in complementary therapies.

The following are potential applications for natural antibiotics in contemporary medicine:

- **Complementary treatment:** Herbal antibiotics can be used with conventional antibiotics as a supplemental treatment to increase the latter's effectiveness. Combining herbal and conventional antibiotics may assist in decreasing the dosage of synthetic antibiotics required, lessen their side effects, and reduce the emergence of resistance.
- **Supporting the Immune System:** Echinacea and astragalus are two common herbal antibiotics with a reputation for strengthening the immune system. By triggering numerous immunological responses, they improve the immune system and assist in warding off diseases.
- **Use as a preventative measure:** Herbal antibiotics with broad-spectrum antibacterial activity include garlic and oregano oil. They might be employed as preventive drugs to stave off infections, particularly when conventional antibiotics are not acceptable or easily accessible.
- **Multi-drug resistant illnesses:** Because multi-drug resistant bacteria are resistant to numerous conventional antibiotics, herbal medications may be especially helpful in treating illnesses brought on by these infections.

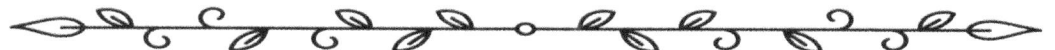

Some herbal antibiotics may work in distinct ways or target bacterial pathways, which could help them overcome resistance mechanisms.

It's crucial to remember that this field of study is still developing, and more research is required to properly grasp herbal antibiotics' potential. To establish their efficacy, safety, and appropriate application in contemporary medicine, rigorous scientific research, clinical trials, and evidence-based data are crucial.

Overall, while the use of conventional antibiotics supported by thorough study and scientific proof continues to be the cornerstone of contemporary medicine, herbal antibiotics have their place in some circumstances.

To ensure responsible and evidence-based incorporation into standard healthcare practices, healthcare practitioners and researchers must interact, share knowledge, and investigate the therapeutic potential of herbal antibiotics.

The Future of Herbal Antibiotics

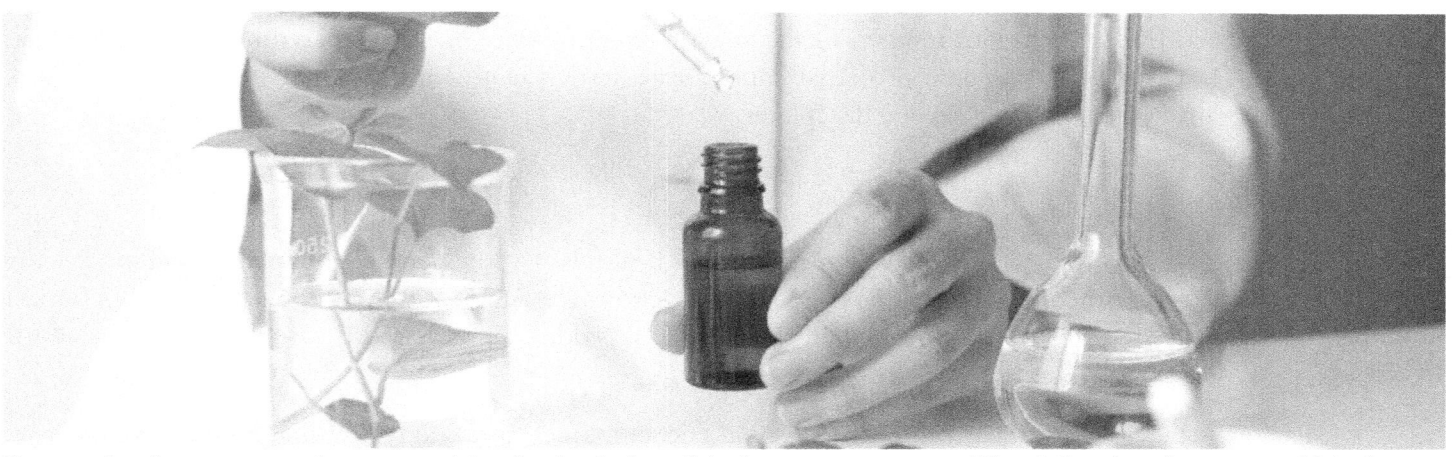

Future developments and opportunities for herbal antibiotics are numerous. The following factors could influence how herbal antibiotics are used in medicine in the future:

1. **Study and Development:** To comprehend the mechanisms of action, identify the active ingredients, and assess the safety and efficacy of herbal antibiotics, an ongoing study is necessary. As additional investigations are undertaken, we can anticipate a greater knowledge of the potential of herbal antibiotics and their use in contemporary medicine.

2. **Targeted Therapies:** With advances in molecular biology and our comprehension of bacterial pathogenesis, it may one day be possible to create herbal antibiotics that directly target virulence factors or vital bacterial pathways. Targeted treatments can lessen interference with healthy micro-biota, lessen adverse effects, and improve overall effectiveness.

3. **Collaboration and Integration:** A more comprehensive approach to healthcare can be achieved by working together with practitioners of traditional medicine, herbalists, naturo-paths, and mainstream healthcare professionals. Herbal antibiotics will become more prevalent in modern medicine by fostering evidence-based practices, knowledge exchange, and bridging gaps between various healthcare systems.

4. **Public Education and Awareness:** It is essential to raise public awareness of the potential of herbal antibiotics and the right way to use them. It will encourage responsible usage and prevent misuse if patients, medical professionals, and the public are informed about herbal antibiotics' advantages, restrictions, and hazards.

5. **The Invention of Novel Herbal Sources:** Exploring new plants, fungi, and creatures for their antimicrobial characteristics can result in the development of novel herbal sources, which can lead to the discovery of new herbal antibiotics. Traditional medical practices from different cultures frequently provide information about medicinal plants that can help researchers find new sources.

6. **Standardization and quality control:** Standardization and quality control are essential for ensuring the consistency of potency and quality of herbal products. The dependability and reproducibility of herbal antibiotics will be improved by establishing standardized extraction techniques, identifying the main active ingredients, and implementing quality control procedures.

7. **Combination therapies:** Adding herbal or traditional or herbal antibiotics to other herbal medicines may improve treatment possibilities. Synergistic interactions between various antibiotics or herbs may improve efficacy, enlarge the range of activity, and reduce the danger of the emergence of resistance.

Herbal antibiotics have a bright future, but to assure their effectiveness, safety, and appropriate use, it is crucial to develop and incorporate them into modern medicine with scientific rigor, evidence-based research, and regulatory monitoring. Harnessing the potential of herbal antibiotics for advancing world healthcare will require continued research and collaboration among several disciplines.

Summary

As more individuals look for safe, natural solutions for their health issues, the herbal antibiotics revolution has drawn major attention. It can potentially change how bacterial infections are handled in the future. However, before these herbal medicines can be widely used, more studies and clinical studies are required to completely understand their efficacy, dose, and safety.

- Patients who cannot tolerate or depend on synthetic antibiotics may find relief using herbal medications.
- Due to their potential for having alternative mechanisms of action and targets from conventional antibiotics, herbal medicines present a fresh approach to fighting infections that have developed resistance.
- Numerous herbal antibiotics have broad-spectrum antibacterial capabilities, which may combat various bacteria, viruses, fungi, and parasites. This adaptability can help in the treatment of different infections.
- Using herbal antibiotics enables synthesizing traditional medical knowledge from diverse civilizations.
- In comparison to synthetic antibiotics, herbal antibiotics may be more environmentally friendly.

Understanding Antibiotic Resistance: A Brief Overview

Antibiotic resistance is not considered a problem by many. But soon, people can be seen to be more and more concerned about their health and what they put in their body. Antibiotics are given to counter an illness that the body has failed to fight with on its own. The body's immune system and gut health should be strong enough to fight small and insignificant illnesses like cough, cold, fever, etc. But there might be a chance that these things elevate and are not combated by the body itself.

While there are options for antibiotics, once the body becomes too used to depending on different traditional medicines, the immunity building inside the body grows weak. There are herbal options that can be taken to stop illnesses from reverting to the body; some herbs also present solutions for preventative measures.

Antibiotic Resistance: Definition

Antibiotic resistance is a serious and growing phenomenon in contemporary medicine and refers to a microorganism's ability to withstand an antibiotic's effects. It is a specific type of drug resistance. Like any other material in the world, if a certain chemical or ingredient is abused, the body may become immune to it.

It is also called antimicrobial resistance, where the bacteria, fungi, parasites, viruses, etc, stop responding to the conventional medication. The medication either fails to treat the diseases completely or it just presents very slow and neglect-able betterment of the disease.

Here's how it works: When bacteria are exposed to antibiotics, most bacteria die or are inhibited. However, some bacteria may survive because they have a characteristic that allows them to resist the antibiotic's effects. These bacteria then multiply, and the next generation may inherit the resistance characteristic, making the antibiotic less effective over time.

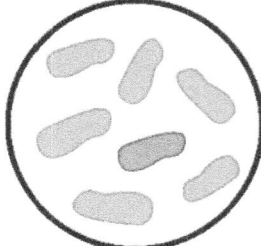
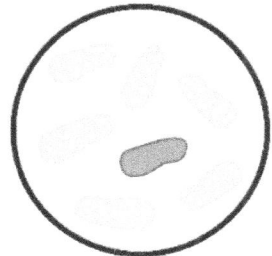
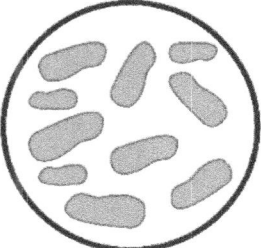
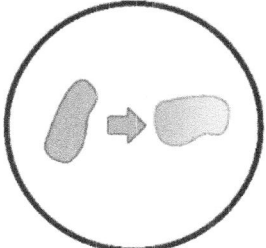

| Lots of germs and some are drug resistant | Antibiotics kill the bacteria causing the illnes as well as the good bacteria protecting the body from infection | The drug resistant bacteria is now able to grow and take over | Some bacteria give their drug resistance to other bacteria |

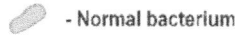 - Normal bacterium   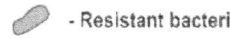 - Resistant bacterium   - Dead bacterium

Antibiotic resistance can naturally occur due to genetic changes in the bacteria, but it is often amplified through the misuse and overuse of antibiotics. This can happen in healthcare settings, in farming practices where animals use antibiotics for growth promotion and disease prevention, and when individuals do not complete their full course of prescribed antibiotics.

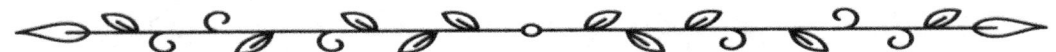

The primary concern with antibiotic resistance is that it can lead to superbug—strains of bacteria resistant to multiple antibiotic types. These superbugs can be extremely difficult to treat, increasing the risk of disease spread, severe illness, and death.

For example, some of the diseases have become resistant to most of the antibiotics that are prevalent in the market. Methicillin-resistant Staphylococcus aureus (MRSA) and multi-drug-resistant Micro-Bacterium tuberculosis (MDR-TB) are two well-known superbug that significantly threaten human health. Two others are also common diseases that often become resistant to antibiotics due to the strength and genetic formation of the bacteria; those diseases are vancomycin-resistant Enterococcus (VRE) and a gut health disease known as Carbapenem-resistant Enterobacteriaceae (CRE).

To combat antibiotic resistance, it is crucial to use antibiotics appropriately and only when prescribed by a healthcare professional. It's also important to invest in research to develop new antibiotics, use diagnostic tests to tailor antibiotic use better, and improve infection control practices.

It is not unknown to mankind when a life is lost to overuse of a drug. Antibiotics are formed using multiple chemicals that may be hard to digest and absorb by a body that is already weak from an illness. If the body does not absorb the antibiotics, it leaves a negative impact on the body and lowers the immunity defense of the body internally.

Antibiotic resistance leads to a lot more complications in the body. The bacteria become stronger and affect other body parts as well, making the body weaker and immune lower. An alternate solution is necessary in the medical field to treat the bacteria. Many complicated cases that require surgeries or chemical radiation cannot be performed without antibiotics.

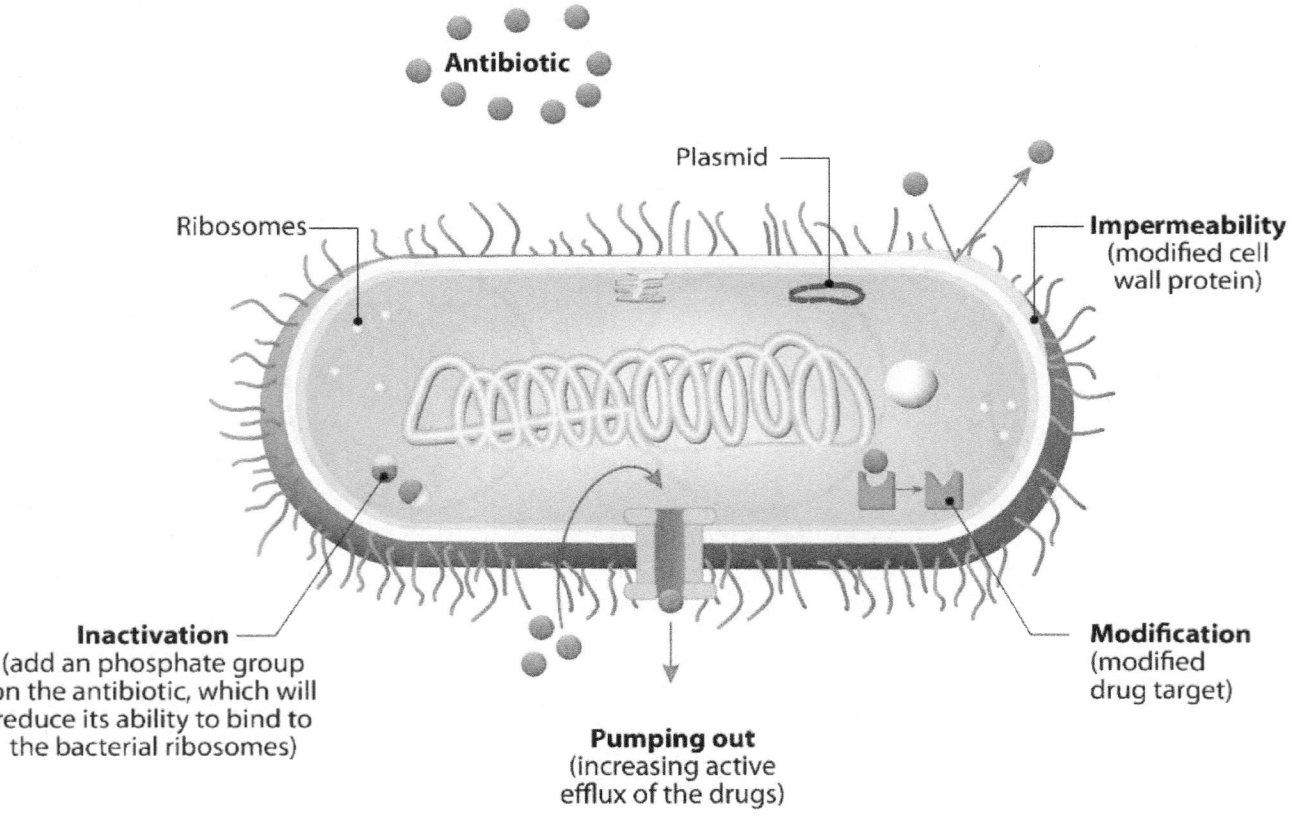

The lower defense mechanism can happen to both humans and animals. Growth of bacteria and no proper treatment present potent risks to the body. These risks are both short-term as well as long-term. Internal damage can be worse

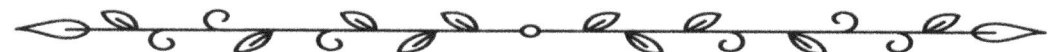

if the bacteria and antibiotics resistance goes neglected. With proper research and acceptable antibiotics from the herbs it is now possible to treat some of the diseases.

The Mechanism of Antibiotic Resistance

Antibiotic resistance is a complex problem, and understanding it requires delving into the realms of microbiology and genetics. A body has bacteria always present. Not all bacteria are bad for health, some bacteria, like in herbal antibiotics it is stated that the bacteria present in yogurt (curd) is a type of bacteria that is good for gut health, and it promotes other good bacteria. Bacteria can develop resistance to antibiotics through several mechanisms:

- **Mutation**: Spontaneous mutations can occur in the bacterial DNA that provide the bacteria with antibiotic resistance. Bacteria that multiply and regenerate pass on the resistance to the next generation. So, it becomes a chain of antibiotic resistant bacteria. When these resistant bacteria multiply, they spread the resistance genes to their offspring. This makes it very less likely for the medication to work on the bacteria or eliminate the disease.
- **Gene Transfer**: Bacteria can also acquire antibiotic resistance genes from other bacteria through a process called horizontal gene transfer (HGT). This can occur through conjugation (direct cell-to-cell transfer), transformation (uptake of DNA from the environment), or transduction (transfer via bacterial viruses, or bacteriophages).

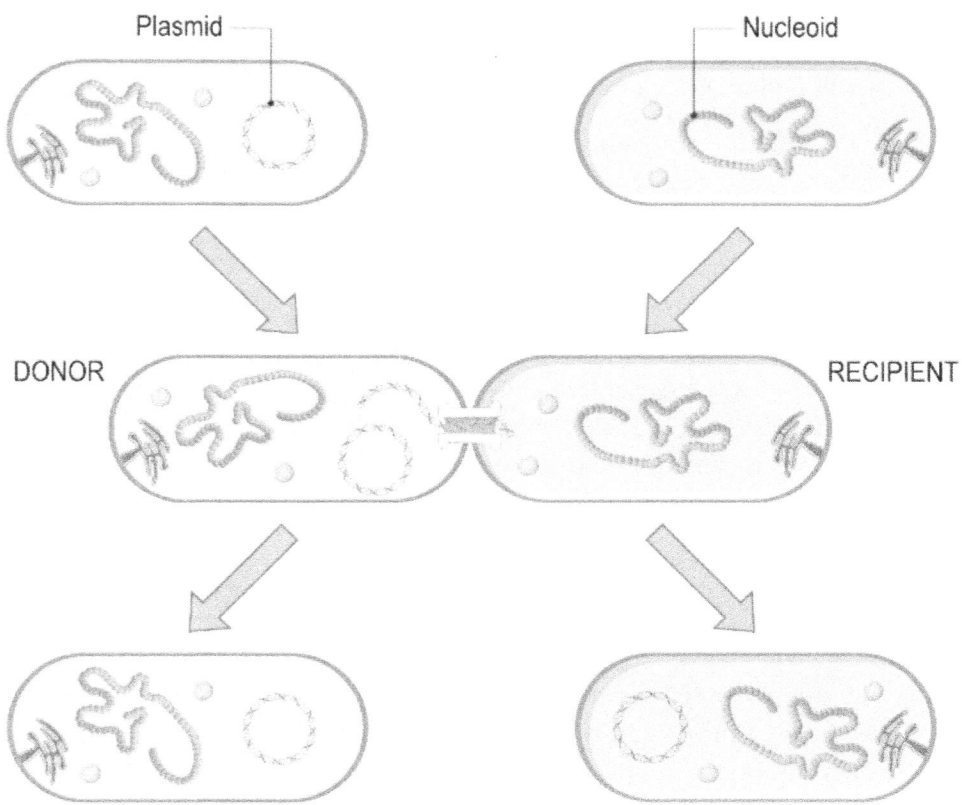

Here are some of the specific ways these genetic changes can result in antibiotic resistance:

A. Altered Target Sites: Antibiotics work by binding to specific target sites in the bacteria, which interferes with the bacterium's ability to function and reproduce. Mutations can change the structure of these target sites so that the antibiotic can no longer bind effectively, rendering it ineffective. For instance, MRSA (methicillin-resistant

Staphylococcus aureus) is resistant to beta-lactam antibiotics because it has acquired a gene (mecA) that produces a modified target protein with lower affinity for these antibiotics. There are many more diseases that occur due to mutation and gene transfer, these processes also change the outlook of the bacteria and the cells containing it. The bacteria which affect only a certain target makes it difficult to treat them with antibiotics, as these bacterial cells feed off healthy cells that are from the antibiotic resistant group.

B. Enzymatic Inactivation or Modification of Antibiotics: Bacteria can produce enzymes that deactivate or modify antibiotics, making them ineffective. For example, beta-lactamases are enzymes that bacteria produce to break the beta-lactam ring, the active site of antibiotics such as penicillin and cephalosporins. Enzymes in a large group modify and change its form to inactivate the antibiotics so that the cells of the disease become immune to the medicine. Enzymatic modification to inactivate antibiotics make it difficult for conventional medicine to work with the cell pattern hence losing its ability to cure the targeted disease.

C. Efflux Pumps: Bacteria can develop proteins that act as efflux pumps, which actively remove antibiotics from the bacterial cell before they can reach their target. Efflux means transporting different compounds out of cells, which includes removing antibiotics from the cells. Once the antibiotics are removed from the cells, before the medication even reaches the target area, it fails to treat the virus or the disease, making the body antibiotic resistant due to efflux pump.

D. Bypassing the Biochemical Pathway: If an antibiotic target a specific metabolic pathway in the bacteria, the bacteria may develop an alternate pathway to bypass the action of the antibiotic. These pathways make the cells undergo changes with enzymes (as discussed earlier in enzymatic inactivation). Once the bacteria pass through the biochemical pathway, it will no longer be affected by the antibiotics.

To combat the issue of antibiotic resistance, scientists are using advanced techniques such as whole-genome sequencing to understand the exact mechanisms of resistance. They are also working on developing new antibiotics, alternatives to antibiotics, and strategies to inhibit resistance mechanisms. For instance, research is being done on the use of efflux pump inhibitors to overcome resistance. They aim to reverse the role of efflux pump and use it in favor of making the cells antibiotic absorbent.

In addition, there is a renewed interest in phage therapy, which uses bacteriophages (viruses that infect bacteria) to treat bacterial infections, and in the use of bacteriocins, proteins produced by bacteria that inhibit the growth of similar or closely related bacterial strains. They are also realizing the role of herbs in making the antibiotic resistant cells revert to their natural mechanism in the natural course of way. Herbal medicines aim to use tools given by nature by extracting and preserving the useful chemicals and using it to the favor of humankind.

Despite these efforts, the development and spread of antibiotic resistance continue to outpace the introduction of new treatments, making this a global public health challenge. Therefore, antibiotic stewardship - ensuring the correct use of antibiotics - and infection control are crucial to prevent the emergence and spread of resistant bacteria.

The research is going two ways, researchers are trying to use the body's ability to turn cells into antibiotic resistant to antibiotic absorbent and on the other hand, natural ingredients are being tested for various diseases and their cures without impacting the cells and their mutation.

The Causes of Antibiotic Resistance

Antibiotic resistance is a major global health concern, occurring when bacteria and other microbes evolve in ways that render the drugs designed to kill them ineffective. This often arises due to the misuse or overuse of antibiotics. There are many other factors also involved in causing antibiotic resistance to the body. The factors are from the internal as well as external environment.

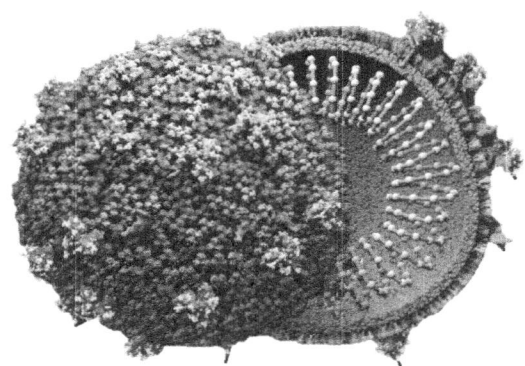

The factors are mainly as those discussed below:

- **Selective Pressure**: Every time a bacterial population is exposed to an antibiotic, it places a selective pressure on it. Bacteria that can survive the antibiotic are able to proliferate, passing on their resistance genes to their offspring and sometimes even other bacteria. This process is a natural consequence of evolution. This also happens due to genes of cells, the new cells that are produced by older cells with antibiotic resistance will not let the antibiotic work as it should on the bacteria.

- **Improper Usage of Antibiotics**: Misuse of antibiotics by not following the full course prescribed or using them for viral infections against which they are ineffective, allows some bacteria to survive and proliferate. Once the doctor prescribes an antibiotic course, it should always run its course on due time, otherwise a side effect is likely to occur. This side effect leads to antibiotic resistance.

- **Overuse in Agriculture and Livestock**: Many farmers use antibiotics not only to treat infections but also as a preventative measure or to promote growth in livestock. This widespread use can lead to a reservoir of antibiotic-resistant bacteria that can spread to humans. Humans consume livestock in many ways, the cells from the livestock effect the internal cell formation within the human body after being consumed. This is a major cause for many countries in Asia banning consumption of poultry fed chicken. Even milk sourced from cows is said to have mutation as most of the cows are fed steroids which alter the cell formation of cows leading to the impact in a human body.

- **Hospital Acquired Infections**: In healthcare settings, where antibiotic use is high, there's a higher chance of resistant bacteria emerging and spreading. With any contact to the things in a clinic or healthcare set-up the chances of transferring such antibiotic resistant bacteria are high.

- **Lack of New Antibiotics**: Drug companies have not been developing as many new antibiotics due to the high costs of development and lower profitability compared to other drugs. This has led to a lack of alternatives when bacteria become resistant to existing antibiotics.

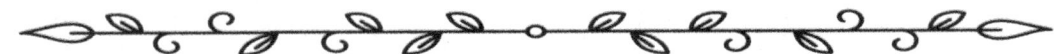

Herbal Antibiotics as Alternate Medication

In the face of increasing antibiotic resistance, there is an urgent need for alternative treatments. One potential source of new antimicrobial agents could be herbal medicines, which have been used for thousands of years to treat a variety of illnesses.

- **Potential of Phyto-chemicals**: Many plants produce secondary metabolites, known as phyto-chemicals, that have antimicrobial properties. These include phenolics, alkaloids, terpenoids, and flavonoid. Research has shown that some of these can be effective against antibiotic-resistant bacteria. These chemicals are in favor of gut health improvement and making the immunity system strong from within.

- **Multi-targeted Approach**: Unlike antibiotics that often have a single target in bacterial cells, phyto-chemicals can affect multiple targets, making it harder for bacteria to develop resistance. These chemicals work on more one targeted area making the body overall stronger and more immune to disease recurrence.

- **Synergistic Effects**: Some herbs can enhance the effects of antibiotics or act synergistic-ally with other herbs to increase their effectiveness. More than one herbs blended make the medicine more powerful and beneficial for health. Many old traditions used garlic, honey, turmeric, onions and many more basic ingredients to treat basic illnesses like; cold and flu at home for young kids and adults alike.

However, there are challenges to using herbal antibiotics as an alternative to conventional ones:

- **Standardization and Quality Control**: The potency of herbal medicines can vary depending on many factors, including the time of harvest, the part of the plant used, and how they are processed. This makes standardization and quality control difficult. The manner to equalize the effects and make the potency similar in all batches, research is still underway. The usefulness of a certain herb or naturally available medicines need to be discovered to uncover the full potential of the available solutions.

- **Safety and Efficacy**: While many plants have a long history of use in traditional medicine, rigorous scientific studies are needed to establish the safety and efficacy of herbal antibiotics. Not all herbs are suitable for all types of bodies like traditional antibiotics. Test and studies need to be performed to determine the adverse effects of certain herbs on certain illnesses that are present in a body being treated for a certain illness. For example, flower extracted honey cannot be given to someone with high blood sugar levels, an alternate herbal medicine will be needed to administer to the person.

- **Regulatory Issues**: Regulatory frameworks for herbal medicines are not as well established as for conventional drugs. This can make it harder for consumers to make informed choices about their use. There is still some time in the research to discover the full potential of available resources.

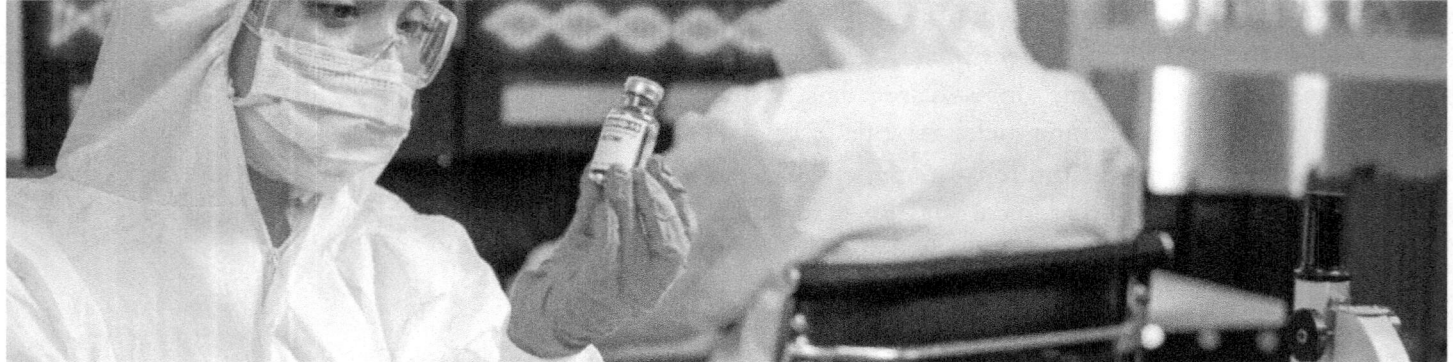

Herbal antibiotics offer potential as an alternative or adjunct treatment to antibiotics. However, more research is

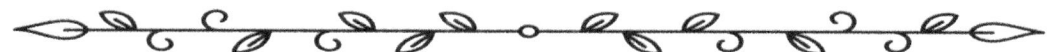

needed to fully understand their mechanisms of action, efficacy, and safety. In a manner like conventional medicine, herbal antibiotics are also in its revolutionary age.

The Impact of Antibiotic Resistance

The impact of antibiotic resistance is profound and far-reaching. If left unchecked, it has the potential to undermine many of the advances in healthcare and medicine that have been achieved over the past century. There is a need to identify and accept a natural course of healing where a slower process which is beneficial in the long run, be given the due importance.

Here are some of the key effects of antibiotic resistance on a personal level:

- **Increased Mortality**: As bacteria become resistant to antibiotics, infections that were once easily treatable can become deadly. According to the World Health Organization, drug-resistant diseases could cause 10 million deaths each year by 2050 if no action is taken. Even small diseases that require a course of antibiotics to treat fully, may become life-threatening if the medication does not perform as per its efficacy.
- **More Complicated Treatments**: Resistant infections often require more extensive medical care, like longer hospital stays, additional tests, and the use of more expensive or toxic medications. This has a lot of negative effects on the health of a person. The longer hospital stays may lead to becoming prone to catching more viruses from other patients. Or toxic medications may lead to organ damage.
- **Compromised Healthcare Procedures**: Antibiotics play a crucial role in many medical procedures, such as surgery, chemotherapy, and organ transplants, where they are used to prevent infections. The rise of antibiotic resistance threatens the safety of these procedures.
- **Increased Healthcare Costs**: The extended hospital stays, and more intensive care required for resistant infections significantly increase healthcare costs. It's estimated that antibiotic resistance could cost the global economy up to $100 trillion by 2050. Not everyone can afford long hospital stays, even on medical insurance, most people cannot take off from work as they must work to fulfil other costs of living.
- **Spread of Infections**: Antibiotic-resistant bacteria can spread from person to person, creating a public health risk. They can also spread in healthcare facilities, posing a risk to vulnerable patients. Having recently come out of a death-trap virus Covid-19, it is now evident how important it is to keep yourself and your family safe from contagious infections.
- **Threat to Global Health Security**: As international travel and trade have become more common, antibiotic resistance has emerged as a global health security threat. Resistant bacteria can quickly spread across borders, and outbreaks can be difficult to control.
- **Return to the Pre-Antibiotic Era**: Without effective antibiotics, we risk returning to the "pre-antibiotic era," when even minor infections could be deadly. This would have profound implications for healthcare, affecting everything from minor surgeries to childbirth. There is an alternate path of herbal antibiotics, which is becoming more important to be researched upon so that it can provide alternate solutions and save the global population from dying of small infections.

Given these impacts, it is crucial to address antibiotic resistance through strategies like improved antibiotic stewardship, infection control, surveillance, and research into new treatments.

The rise of antibiotic resistance has major implications for the medical industry, affecting healthcare providers, pharmaceutical companies, and the broader healthcare system. Below are some of the impacts and consequences:

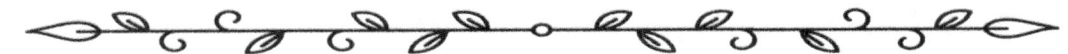

Healthcare Providers:

- **Increased Clinical Complexity**: Antibiotic resistance complicates the treatment of common infections, making them harder to manage. This can result in longer hospital stays and increased mortality rates.
- **Increased Resource Use**: Resistant infections require more resources to treat, from additional tests to identify the resistant strain to more expensive or toxic drugs. This can strain already limited healthcare resources.
- **Increased Risk for Healthcare Workers**: Resistant bacteria can spread in healthcare settings, potentially putting healthcare workers at risk of infection. In the long run it can affect the turnout of future medical persons due to high health risk.

Pharmaceutical Companies:

- **Market Failure for Antibiotics**: The economic model for antibiotic development is challenging. New antibiotics are meant to be used sparingly to preserve their effectiveness, but this limits potential profits and di-incentivizes investment in research and development. This is a setback as well as waste of resources.
- **Pressure to Develop New Drugs**: As resistance grows, there is increasing pressure on pharmaceutical companies to develop new antibiotics. However, the discovery and development of new antibiotics is scientifically challenging, time-consuming, and costly. Not every antibiotic is suitable for every person.

Healthcare System and Industry:

- **Increased Healthcare Costs**: The costs associated with antibiotic resistance are substantial, including longer hospital stays, more intensive care, and the use of more expensive drugs. This places a significant financial burden on healthcare systems. The costs are high, and the funds are limited, costs need to be cut down and funds need to be allocated sensibly to tick all the boxes.
- **Impact on Medical Procedures**: Many medical procedures and treatments, including surgeries, chemotherapy, and organ transplants, rely on antibiotics to prevent infections. The rise of antibiotic resistance threatens the safety and effectiveness of these procedures. Once a body produces cells that become resistant to antibiotics, it becomes almost impossible to perform a certain medical procedure on the body.
- **Regulatory Challenges**: Regulatory agencies face challenges in encouraging the development of new antibiotics and ensuring their appropriate use. They also play a role in monitoring and controlling the spread of resistant bacteria. This process is time consuming and expensive. Circulating a medicine and then calling it back has and can cause a cost of millions of dollars.

In addition to these impacts, the rise of antibiotic resistance can also have broader societal consequences, such as inhibiting progress in healthcare, reducing the population's trust in the medical industry, and posing a threat to global public health security. As such, it is a problem that requires a coordinated, global response involving not only the medical industry but also policymakers, researchers, and the public.

Growth in the prevalence of herbal antibiotics as an alternate solution is proposing hope to the medical industry all around the world. Many old concoctions and medicines made from herbs are being tested under the light of technology to unveil the truth.

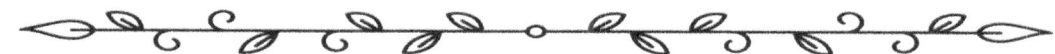

Combating Antibiotic Resistance

Combating antibiotic resistance is a complex challenge that requires a multifaceted approach involving various sectors and stakeholders. Here are several strategies being implemented or proposed to address the issue, all these strategies will be discussed in detail in the chapters to come, here is a brief overview of each strategy:

- **Stewardship Programs**: Antibiotic stewardship programs involve coordinated interventions designed to improve and measure the appropriate use of antibiotics. This includes ensuring that antibiotics are only used, when necessary, that the right drug is selected, and that it is given at the right dose and for the right duration. To ensure this, it is important to consult a doctor or a medical practitioner.

- **Infection Prevention and Control**: By preventing infections, the need for antibiotics can be reduced. Infection prevention measures include effective hand hygiene, vaccination, safe food preparation, and using antibiotics responsibly in agriculture and livestock. This is a collective effort of a nation. Anyone sector cannot make it work, or even one sector lagging can cause this strategy to fail miserably.

- **Surveillance and Monitoring**: Surveillance systems track antibiotic resistance trends and antibiotic use in human health and agriculture. This data can be used to guide interventions, monitor their effectiveness, and provide an early warning of emerging resistance. An early warning can be used to perform alternate medications to treat the illness without letting it become fatal.

- **Research and Development of New Antibiotics**: Given the emergence of multi-drug resistant bacteria, there is an urgent need for new antibiotics. This includes incentive's pharmaceutical companies to invest in antibiotic research and development, despite the challenging economic model. On the other hand, it is also important to recognize herbal antibiotics as an alternate path to achieve the goal of a healthy global population.

- **Development of Alternatives to Antibiotics**: There is growing interest in alternative therapies, such as phage therapy, probiotics, immunotherapies, and vaccines, that could reduce the reliance on antibiotics. Probiotics and other supplements are being given from a young age to get most out of the strategy in the long run.

- **Public Education**: Increasing public awareness about the risks of antibiotic resistance and the importance of using antibiotics responsibly is critical. This includes educating patients not to demand antibiotics for viral infections, and to always complete the full course of antibiotics when they are prescribed. Apart from large scale industry, each person is responsible for making sure that they play their part of not abusing antibiotics.

- **Regulation and Policy**: Governments and international organizations can play a key role by implementing regulations to ensure the responsible use of antibiotics, encouraging the development of new drugs, and coordinating global efforts to combat antibiotic resistance.

- **One Health Approach**: Antibiotic resistance is a problem that crosses human, animal, and environmental health. Therefore, a "One Health" approach that coordinates efforts across these sectors is essential. It is an effort at a global level regardless of the monetary and economic state of different countries, each country needs to step up and play their role.

These efforts will need to be sustained over the long term and coordinated globally, as antibiotic resistance is a problem that knows no borders. Despite the challenges, with concerted effort, it is possible to combat antibiotic resistance and safeguard the effectiveness of antibiotics for future generations. This along with the implementation of herbal antibiotics at a larger scale will promise a healthy world now and forever.

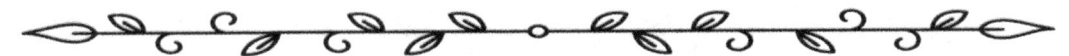

Summary

Herbal antibiotics are a promising substitute to conventional antibiotics where there is antibiotic resistance. Research is being conducted and more people are shifting their mindset from traditional medication to herbal options.

While there is still no promise of a treatment for each illness, there still is hope with both traditional as well as herbal medicines together.

We can gather a lot of important notes from this chapter about understanding antibiotic resistance:

- Antibiotic resistance is when the cells in a body mutate, and the antibiotic being administered becomes ineffective on the bacteria due to the cell's mutation.
- The cells also pass on the resistance to the new cells being generated in the body, through gene transfer, which makes it more difficult to counter a disease using antibiotics.
- Causes of antibiotic resistance include; abuse of antibiotics, not using the antibiotics as per the doctor's recommendation, selective pressure of bacteria due to gene transfer in cells, overuse of antibiotics and steroids in livestock and agriculture, etc.
- Herbal antibiotics present an alternate solution to some of the diseases. The phyto-chemicals are known to target more than one area making it difficult for the bacteria to spread or attack the cells. There are challenges with herbal antibiotics as well, like; lack of standardization, safety and efficiency of the antibiotic, etc.
- There are many negative impacts of antibiotic resistance in humans, some of these impacts are higher mortality rate, higher cost of medication, longer and complex medical procedures to combat an illness, etc.
- Strategies can be implemented to combat antibiotic resistance, some of the strategies are; stewardship programs, development of alternate solutions such as herbal antibiotics, surveillance and monitoring.

Power of Nature:
an Introduction to Herbal Antibiotics

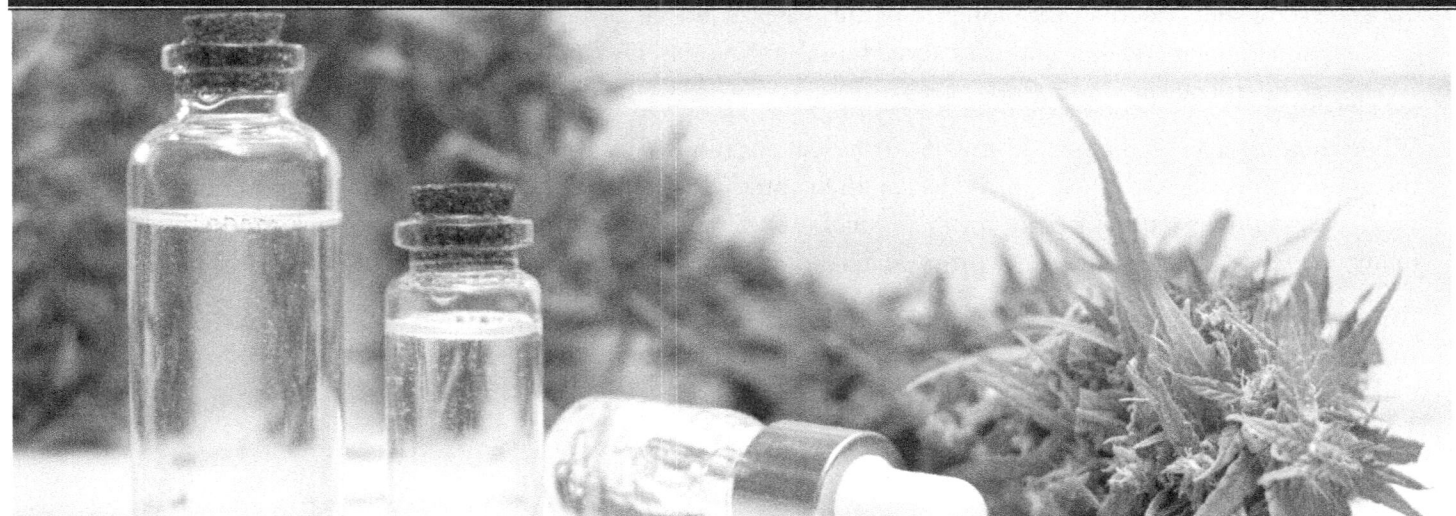

Herbal antibiotics refer to plant-based substances that can inhibit the growth of or destroy different forms of negatively impacting cells like; bacteria, fungi, viruses, or parasites, much like conventional antibiotics. These plant-based antibiotics are usually derived from various parts of plants including roots, leaves, bark, and fruit, and have been used for centuries in traditional medicine around the world to treat various ailments.

Herbal antibiotics have not been in the form you see them today since its evolution. These were made in rough form by grinding the herbs by hand in a mortar and pestle or just crushing by stone. Some parts of the plans were taken and then medicines and even ointments were made using the plants and herbs to treat various illnesses and even poisonous bites of different animals and reptiles.

Traditional antibiotics have mainly depended on chemical formations and making medicines by mixing a few or many chemicals and even gases together and then the researchers would experiment and study the medicine to make sure its use and effectiveness. While both antibiotics are based on trial and error after deep and tiring study, there are many differences between the two forms of treatment. The main difference between herbal antibiotics and traditional (conventional) medicine lies in their origin and the approach to treating diseases.

- **Origin**: Conventional antibiotics are typically synthesized in laboratories, often initially inspired by natural substances but then modified and standardized for mass production. They usually consist of a single active compound that targets a specific bacterial function or structure. On the other hand, herbal antibiotics are derived directly from plants and often comprise a complex mix of compounds that can work together. Herbal antibiotics also largely depend on the availability of the plants and herbs, and it may be only available in a certain season while traditional medicines are created using synthetic chemicals which are mostly processed by humans.

- **Approach to Treating Diseases**: Conventional medicine tends to focus on treating symptoms or targeting specific pathogens, often using a "one size fits all" approach. Herbal medicine, however, takes a more holistic approach, looking at the entire individual and their overall health. Herbal antibiotics may also have multiple modes of action due to their complex mixture of compounds. (As discussed earlier in chapter 2) Herbal antibiotics are multitarget agents, they focus on the bacteria and make it weak and not let it spread to other areas.

- **Side Effects**: Conventional antibiotics can sometimes lead to side effects such as digestive issues or antibiotic resistance when used frequently or improperly. Herbal antibiotics, while not free of potential side effects, are often seen as a more natural and gentler alternative, though they may be less potent.
- **Regulation and Standardization**: Conventional antibiotics are strictly regulated, with dosages and uses well established. Herbal antibiotics, on the other hand, are often not as tightly regulated, which can lead to variability in quality and efficacy. Herbal antibiotics also need more time and study to make sure of its standardization.

While there is growing interest in the use of herbal antibiotics, it's important to note that they should be used under the supervision of a healthcare provider, as their interactions with other medications and potential side effects can vary. Despite their natural origin, they can still be potent and potentially harmful if used improperly. Further, while many plant-based substances show promise in laboratory settings, their effectiveness in human bodies can vary widely.

Another major concern arises with weather and climate suitability of the desired plant or herb. Not every season is suitable for each herb or plant needed to make a certain medicine.

History of Herbal Antibiotics

The history of herbal antibiotics is vast and diverse, stretching back thousands of years across numerous cultures. It's a testament to humankind's enduring relationship with nature and our instinctive drive to seek healing from our surroundings. There has been evidence of people without having any scientific knowledge tried to find, cure and heal their illnesses and diseases with the help of plants and herbs available to them locally.

In the earliest days of human existence, healing likely started as trial and error. Prehistoric humans observed animals and noted which plants they used when they were ill. They experimented with those plants themselves, discovered their therapeutic properties, and passed the knowledge down through generations.

- Cave paintings dating back to 6000 BC hint at the use of plants as medicine.
- In the ancient world, herbal medicine was considered a mainstay of healthcare. In Egypt, the Ebers Papyrus, dated to around 1550 BC, details the medicinal use of over 700 plants, including garlic, juniper, and cannabis. They even used myrrh and honey, both known for their antimicrobial properties, in wound care.
- Ancient China also made significant contributions to herbal medicine. The legendary Emperor Shen Nong, said to have lived around 2800 BC, is credited with cataloging hundreds of medicinal plants in the "Shen Nong Ben Cao Jing" (The Divine Farmer's Materia Medica). This work became the foundation of Traditional Chinese Medicine, which heavily relies on herbal therapies even today.
- In the subcontinent of Asia, (present-day India and Pakistan), the ancient practice of Ayurveda (meaning "knowledge of life" in Sanskrit), dating back to 1500 BC, employs a vast variety of plants for their healing properties. Turmeric, neem, and tulsi are just a few examples of herbs used in Ayurveda medicine with known antibiotic properties.
- In Europe, the Greeks and Romans had an extensive knowledge of medicinal plants. Hippocrates, the "Father of Medicine," documented the medicinal use of about 400 plants. Dioscorides, a Greek physician in the first century AD, wrote "De Materia Medica," a five-volume encyclopedia about herbal medicine and related medicinal substances, which was widely read for more than 1,500 years.

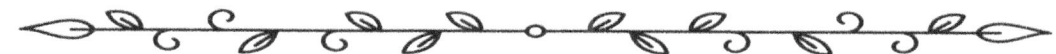

How did Pharmacology come into being?

The Middle Ages saw the growth of herbal gardens in monasteries, where monks preserved and expanded the knowledge of medicinal plants. During the Renaissance, herbal medicine became more systematized, and the understanding of the medicinal properties of plants expanded, with the publication of many herbals – books describing the properties and uses of plants.

The use of plants as medicine continued to prevail until the 19th century when scientists began isolating active ingredients from plants, thus marking the beginning of modern pharmacology.

One key example is the isolation of salicin from willow bark, leading to the creation of aspirin. With multiple examples present in the modern-day medicine, it is important to keep herbal medicines in sync with conventional medicines to make the most out of both the studies.

Despite this shift towards synthetic drugs, the World Health Organization estimates that nearly 80% of the world's population still relies on herbal medicines for part of their primary healthcare. It's a practice that remains especially prevalent in developing countries, where access to synthetic drugs can be limited. It is also due to reliance and ease of availability of good quality herbs to the nations that most of the population chooses herbal medication over conventional medicines for treating minor diseases.

In recent decades, there's been a resurgence of interest in herbal antibiotics in the Western world, driven by increasing concerns about antibiotic resistance. Scientists are now looking back to traditional medicines in the search for new antimicrobial agents. Numerous studies are ongoing to scientifically validate the antibiotic properties of various medicinal plants and explore ways to use them to fight resistant bacteria.

The history of herbal antibiotics is as old as humanity itself. These natural remedies have sustained and nurtured us, acting as our allies in the fight against disease. As we face new health challenges, it seems increasingly likely that we will continue to turn to these ancient resources for solutions.

The herbal antibiotics are here to stay, so it is important and inevitable that research and formulae are made with herbs and plants so that reliable antibiotics can be invented. This will also lead to lesser antibiotic resistance in the body by the bacteria and help prevent mutation of cells and gene transfer.

Together, both the antibiotics, conventional and herbal, can help the world in a great manner to overcome a lot of fatal diseases. Allotting proper resources to research and the cost of the experiment may be higher but the studies are worth it as it will benefit humankind for a long term and many generations to come.

How Herbal Antibiotics Work?

Herbal antibiotics work similarly to synthetic antibiotics in that they aim to inhibit the growth of bacteria or kill them outright. The main target is to combat the bacteria that is the main cause of the disease of the illness. However, unlike conventional antibiotics that often have a single active compound targeting a specific bacterial function or structure, herbal antibiotics often contain multiple active compounds that can have a variety of effects, potentially targeting several different aspects of bacterial physiology at once.

Herbal antibiotics use a complex mix of several herbs and parts of different plants to make one medicine. These parts and herbs have a natural capability to treat a lot of things at one time. Apart from medication purpose, herbs have also been used and are still used by the beauty industry as there are multiple herbs and plants known to humankind that aid healthy skin, even skin texture and even hair growth.

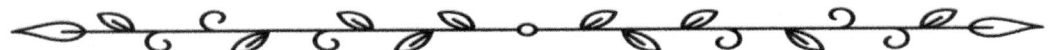

Herbs are a gift of nature that contain power to heal and even finish a disease from the root cause if used properly. Plants and parts of plants known to humankind have different chemicals that benefits the healing process, the process maybe slow but it is effective in the long run.

Here's a general look at how herbal antibiotics can work:

- **Inhibiting Bacterial Growth**: Some plant compounds can inhibit bacterial growth by interfering with critical processes such as protein synthesis, cell wall synthesis, or nucleic acid synthesis. This is like the action of conventional antibiotics. The compounds prevent the bacteria from spreading to other parts and even help degenerate the bacteria cells.

- **Directly Killing Bacteria**: Certain plant compounds have bactericidal properties, meaning they can kill bacteria directly. This can occur through various mechanisms, such as disrupting the bacterial cell membrane, leading to leakage of vital cellular contents. Some chemicals in plants and herbs are poisonous for bacterial cells in the body. This is why they can kill the bacteria and finish the disease in a manner that is not possible by conventional medicine.

- **Boosting the Immune System**: Many plants have properties that can stimulate the body's immune system, enhancing its ability to fight off bacterial infections. This is a somewhat indirect form of antibiotic activity, as it involves boosting the body's natural defenses rather than directly targeting the bacteria. Herbal antibiotics have herbs that help build a stronger immunity system so that in the future, the body can produce cells that fight the disease on its own without requiring antibiotics.

- **Antioxidant Effects**: Some plants have potent antioxidant properties. By neutralizing harmful free radicals in the body, these plants can help to maintain the optimal function of the immune system and other physiological processes that are involved in resisting bacterial infections. The chemicals from the plants make the body strong internally and it can function without having external support of medicine. Other harmful bacteria are also aimed by the herbal antibiotics, making the antibiotics useful to stay healthy for a longer period.

- **Synergistic Effects**: Herbal remedies often involve mixtures of different plants, and there can be synergistic effects between the various plant compounds. This can result in greater overall antimicrobial activity than would be seen with the individual compounds alone. Unlike, conventional antibiotics where a single compound is the main ingredient, herbal antibiotics is based on multiple active ingredients, making it more potent and effective.

- **Disrupting Quorum Sensing**: Some plant compounds can interfere with quorum sensing, a system of stimulus and response correlated to population density among bacteria. By disrupting this communication, plants can hinder the bacteria's ability to form biofilms, coordinate defenses, and express virulence factors, thereby reducing their ability to establish and maintain infections.

It's important to note that while many plant compounds have been shown to have antimicrobial activity in laboratory settings, their effectiveness in the human body can be affected by various factors, including how they're prepared and administered, their absorption and metabolism in the body, and the presence of other compounds in the body.

Therefore, while herbal antibiotics can certainly be beneficial, they should be used judiciously and preferably under the guidance of a healthcare provider. The herbal antibiotics also have a greater effect of the weather and climate compared to the conventional antibiotics.

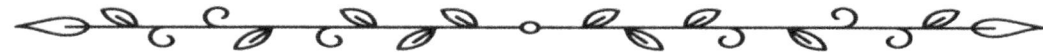

The Benefits of Herbal Antibiotics

The use of herbal antibiotics has been recognized for thousands of years in traditional medicine, and recent scientific research has started to validate some of these ancient practices.

Herbal antibiotics are few and still are in the evolutionary period, but the ones that are present have proven to be helpful in curing the ailment. There are multiple benefits of herbal antibiotics known to science. One of the major benefits is that it aims at multiple areas. So, the bacteria, if spreading, will not be able to affect more areas or organs of the body due to the complex compound of ingredients present in the herbal antibiotics. Here are some potential benefits of using herbal antibiotics:

- **Effectiveness Against Antibiotic-Resistant Bacteria**: One of the most promising aspects of herbal antibiotics is their potential effectiveness against antibiotic-resistant bacteria. Many plant compounds have been found to be effective against these so-called "superbugs" in laboratory studies. Some plant compounds can even enhance the effectiveness of conventional antibiotics or interfere with mechanisms of antibiotic resistance. However, much more research is needed to fully understand and utilize these effects in a clinical setting. In near future, the era of herbal antibiotics looks promising.

- **Fewer Side Effects**: Herbal antibiotics are often considered to be gentler on the body than synthetic antibiotics, with fewer side effects. For example, they are less likely to disrupt the gut micro-biota, a common issue with conventional antibiotics that can lead to problems like diarrhea and yeast infections. However, herbal remedies are not completely devoid of side effects and can interact with other medications, so they should be used with care. The compound of herbal antibiotics should be such that it doesn't impact other things negatively.

- **Holistic Health**: Herbal medicine often takes a more holistic approach to health, aiming to promote overall well-being rather than just treating specific symptoms or diseases. Many medicinal plants have multiple health benefits beyond their antimicrobial activity, such as anti-inflammatory, antioxidant, or immune-boosting effects, which can contribute to this holistic health benefit. One antibiotic will render multiple benefits to the body at the same time. This is not likely the case with conventional antibiotics. Rather conventional antibiotics can cause other diseases to treat one disease at hand.

- **Accessibility and Sustainability**: Many medicinal plants can be grown locally and sustainably, making them more accessible and potentially more affordable than conventional antibiotics, particularly in low-income regions. This can also have environmental benefits, as sustainable cultivation of medicinal plants can contribute to biodiversity and carbon sequestration. Herbal antibiotics are not only serving a human body, but they are also beneficial for the Eco-system. Planting certain herbs and plants to be available locally means that more trees and greenery will be present at multiple locations.

- **Complementary Action**: Herbal antibiotics typically contain a multitude of active compounds, which can have a broader spectrum of activity compared to conventional antibiotics that typically have a single active ingredient. This multifaceted approach can potentially be more effective in treating complex or persistent infections. Apart from this, the multifaceted approach also helps with the immunity. Once the body becomes capable of fighting a certain bacterium, the chances of falling ill to those same bacteria again are slim.

- **Preventive Medicine**: Many medicinal plants not only help in fighting off existing infections but also have a role in preventive healthcare due to their immune-boosting properties. This aligns with the principle of preventive medicine, focusing on maintaining health and preventing disease rather than just treating disease. This is a huge benefit, keeping in mind its long-term effects. The bacteria killed will not be able to recur due to the immunity being strong.

Despite these potential benefits, it's important to note that herbal antibiotics should be used judiciously and under the supervision of a healthcare provider. While many plant compounds have shown promising antimicrobial activity in laboratory studies, clinical evidence is still limited, and factors such as dosage, preparation, and individual differences in absorption and metabolism can all affect their effectiveness in practice.

Further research is needed to fully understand the potential of herbal antibiotics and to develop guidelines for their safe and effective use. With research and experimentation, safe and standardized antibiotics can be made available to cure different diseases that currently only rely on conventional medication.

Common Misconceptions about Herbal Antibiotics

There are several misconceptions about herbal antibiotics that can lead to misuse or unrealistic expectations. Here are some common ones:

- **"All Herbal Antibiotics are Safe Because They're Natural"**: While it's true that herbal antibiotics are derived from natural sources, this doesn't automatically make them safe. Like any medicine, they can have side effects, especially when taken in large amounts or combined with other substances. They can also trigger allergies in some people.
- **"Herbal Antibiotics Work Just Like Synthetic Antibiotics"**: While some herbal antibiotics can kill bacteria or inhibit their growth, their mechanisms of action can be very different from those of synthetic antibiotics. Herbal remedies often contain a variety of active compounds that can have a range of effects on the body, not all of which are directly related to fighting bacteria. There are both pros and cons of having such a complex compound in your body especially if you are unaware of its true potential.
- **"Herbal Antibiotics are Effective Against All Types of Infections"**: Just like synthetic antibiotics, different herbal remedies are effective against different types of bacteria, and not all are effective against all types of infections.
- **"Herbal Antibiotics Can Replace Synthetic Antibiotics in All Cases"**: While herbal antibiotics can be a valuable tool in the fight against bacterial infections, they should not be seen as a replacement for synthetic antibiotics in all cases. For severe or life-threatening infections, synthetic antibiotics are often the best choice, due to their potency and the extensive clinical evidence supporting their use. Herbal antibiotics can be a useful complement to conventional treatment or an alternative in cases where conventional antibiotics cannot be used, but they are not a cure-all.
- **"Herbal Antibiotics Do Not Require Professional Guidance"**: While many people self-prescribe herbal antibiotics, it's essential to use them under the guidance of a healthcare provider. Dosage, preparation, and potential interactions with other medications are all important considerations that a professional can help with.

While herbal medicine offers a lot of potential, it's important to approach it with an informed and balanced view, understanding both its strengths and limitations. Properly used, herbal antibiotics can be a valuable part of our toolkit for maintaining health and fighting disease. Granting an immeasurable chance of curing diseases across the globe.

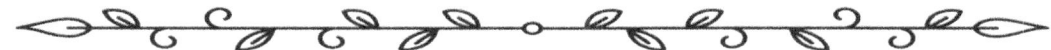

Summary

Herbal antibiotics is the natures gift to mankind. The herbal antibiotics can treat multiple ailments, but it also presents some cons to the humankind. Here is a quick glance at what we have covered in this chapter:

- Herbal antibiotics are extractions and complex compounds made from herbs and parts of plants.
- Herbal antibiotics and conventional synthetic antibiotics are not similar, and they do not work in a similar pattern. Both have different origin, and the safety and dosage are also different from each other. The safety protocol of both antibiotics is very different.
- It is as old as mankind itself that herbs and plants are used to treat sick and use as preventative tools. In the 19th century, scientists started using herbs to form conventional medicine keeping only one active ingredient in the medicine instead of a complex mix of chemicals. This was the start of Pharmacology.
- There are some misconceptions about herbal antibiotics. Even though it is mainly sourced from natures resources, it is not a natural remedy. Herbal antibiotics also need supervision and dosage prescription from a certified and trained professional. The herbal antibiotics cannot be self-prescribed, it can result in a disastrous outcome.

Sustainable and Ethical Herb Gathering

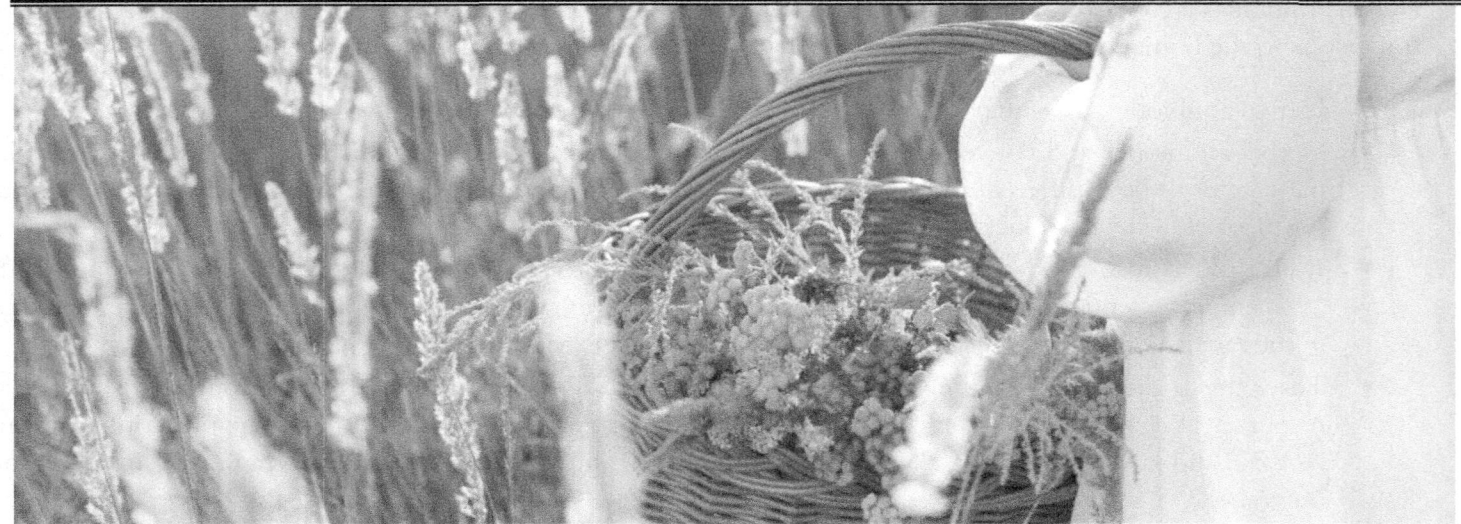

Herb gathering that is sustainable and ethical involves picking herbs to protect the environment's long-term health and local communities' well-being. It entails monitoring harvesting procedures to make sure that neither herb populations nor the ecosystems to which they belong are harmed. Instead, gatherers want to encourage biodiversity, safeguard endangered species, and permit plant regrowth through natural means.

Gatherers must be aware of the plants they collect and their native habitats to accomplish sustainable and ethical herb gathering. They must abide by local rules and ordinances, obtain appropriate permissions, and refrain from over-harvesting. Fair-trade principles should also be used to ensure equitable pay for gatherers and support community-based projects.

We can ensure that medicinal and culinary herbs are available for future generations, safeguard the delicate exosystemic balance, and promote the welfare of regional people who rely on these resources by engaging in sustainable and ethical herb collection.

The Importance of Sustainability in Herb Gathering

The sustainability of herb collection is crucial because it guarantees the ongoing availability of these natural resources while preserving the well-being of communities and ecosystems. Here are some main arguments in favor of the necessity of sustainability in herb gathering:

Biodiversity conservation: Sustainable methods of gathering herbs aid in the protection of the biodiversity of plants. Gatherers avoid over-exploitation of species and support a healthy environment by taking only a small portion of the available herbs and allowing for natural regeneration. In turn, this promotes the overall stability and health of ecosystems and aids in preserving biodiversity.

Preservation of traditional knowledge: Sustainable herb collection techniques aid in preserving traditional plant knowledge. Numerous indigenous groups possess important knowledge regarding the therapeutic and traditional uses of plants. By harvesting these herbs sustainably, we can ensure that this knowledge is passed down through the generations and not lost over time.

Mitigation of the environmental impact: Illegal methods of obtaining herbs might negatively influence the ecosystem. Certain plant species may deteriorate or become extinct due to over-harvesting. In addition, toxic chemicals

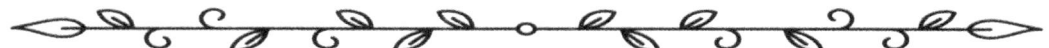

or destructive methods can affect ecosystems and upset the delicate balance of habitats. Gatherers reduce their environmental effects and safeguard the health of ecosystems by implementing sustainable practices.

Adaptation to climate change: Sustainable herb collection techniques can help in decreasing the effects of climate change. Many plants have therapeutic qualities that can help alleviate some health ailments linked to climate change, such as respiratory conditions or illnesses brought on by stress. We can keep access to these priceless resources and increase our ability to withstand climate change by ensuring that herb gathering is sustainable.

Opportunities for the economy: Local communities can make money by picking herbs. Gatherers can guarantee the durability of this economic opportunity by practicing sustainability. Sustainable practices enable a constant supply of herbs, sustaining the livelihoods of those engaged in herb collection rather than diminishing resources.

Sustainability in herb collection is essential to retain biodiversity, safeguard ecosystems, maintain traditional knowledge, promote local economies, reduce environmental impact, and adapt to the difficulties posed by climate change. By engaging in sustainable herb collection, we can ensure by following the right guidelines, that future generations continue to have access to and benefit from these priceless natural resources.

On the other hand, some handful issues can't be ignored during herb gatherings. Significant problems with herb gathering include over-harvesting and the destruction of habitats. Herbs are over-harvested when gathered in excess, frequently faster than they naturally regenerate. This can cause some plant species to decrease or possibly go extinct, upsetting the delicate balance of ecosystems.

Another issue is habitat degradation, as actions such as picking herbs can harm or destroy the natural environments in which these plants thrive. The targeted herb species, the larger ecosystem, and the species that depend on it might be harmed by clearing land, trampling vegetation, and damaging harvesting techniques.

Herb collection methods that are ethical and sustainable are crucial to addressing these problems. This entails using regenerative harvesting methods, such as simply taking a small fraction of the available herbs and letting them regenerate naturally. It is also part of utilizing non-destructive harvesting techniques, respecting protected areas, and taking action to lessen environmental impact.

Gatherers must be aware of the value of sustainable practices and the potential repercussions of over-harvesting and habitat loss. Furthermore, putting in place laws and rules that encourage sustainable collection and safeguard habitats can aid in resolving these problems on a bigger scale.

Understanding Ethical Herb Gathering

Before diving more into this chapter, we should clearly understand what ethical herb gathering is. Understanding ethical herb gathering is essential to learn about herb gathering in general. So, moving forward, we will first learn about the basics of ethical herb gathering.

Herb gathering that abides by the ideals of justice, sustainability, and awareness of one's impact on the environment and surrounding communities is known as ethical herb gathering. It also considers the social and cultural components beyond merely ensuring ecological sustainability. The following are the main components to understand the concept of ethical herb gathering:

- **Respect for neighborhood communities:** Ethical herb collectors are aware of and respect the rights, wisdom, and customs of the local communities with a long history of working with herbs. They form cooperative alliances, seek advice from local authorities, and ensure that herb collection's advantages are distributed fairly.

- **Fair-trade and just compensation:** Ethical herb gathering incorporates fair-trade procedures that guarantee gatherers receive just compensation and respectable working circumstances. This makes it easier for those who harvest herbs, especially those who live in under-served or indigenous communities, to build a stable and respectable income.

- **Cultural sensitivity:** For some local populations, the collecting of herbs may have ceremonial, spiritual, or cultural importance. By obtaining consent and following culturally relevant protocol, ethical gatherers respect these customs and cultural practices related to the herbs.

- **Wild population sustainability:** It is a top priority for ethical herb gatherers, who emphasize the longevity and quantity of wild herb populations. They follow harvesting procedures that support the continued survival and vitality of the plants they gather because they are aware of their life cycles and patterns of regeneration.

- **Environmental responsibility:** Ethical collection methods reduce their negative effects on the environment. This entails merely taking what is required, employing non-destructive methods, preventing habitat loss, and safeguarding rare or endangered plant species.

- **Transparency and traceability:** Ethical gatherers ensure their methods are transparent by disclosing details about the location, standard, and longevity of the herbs they give. Additionally, they keep traceable records, which aids in monitoring and assessing their operations' environmental and social effects.

- **Education and empowerment:** They are top priorities for ethical herb gatherers, both in their communities and among consumers. They enable others to make educated decisions and encourage ethical herb-gathering practices by spreading awareness of the value of sustainability and cultural preservation.

An all-encompassing strategy that considers social, cultural, economic, and environmental concerns is required for ethical herb collection. Herb gatherers can support the long-term supply of medicinal and culinary herbs while preserving biodiversity, cultural legacy, and community well-being by upholding ethical standards.

We should also have an intense awareness of the environment and a dedication to protecting it are necessary for ethical herb collection that respects nature and considers future generations' needs. Herbs are picked in a way that promotes ecosystem health and allows for their regeneration since gatherers prioritize sustainable practices. Ethical gatherers aim to guarantee the long-term availability of these priceless resources, preserving them for years to come by considering future generations' requirements.

Principles of Sustainable and Ethical Herb Gathering

We cannot understand sustainable and ethical herb gathering unless we know and learn the key principles and guidelines regarding sustainable and ethical herb gathering. To ensure the vital health and sustainability of plant populations and ecosystems, sustainable and ethical herb harvesting entails the careful and courteous harvest of plants for medicinal, culinary, or spiritual purposes means that without learning the fundamental principles, we can't learn the core concept of sustainable and ethical herb gathering.

The following guiding principles can help you pick herbs ethically and ecologically:

- One of the most crucial tenets of sustainable herb harvesting is the treatment of the plants we pick with respect and gratitude. Because they can cure us, plants should be treated with respect and gratitude. Rituals, prayers, or simply pausing to thank the plant before harvesting can accomplish this.

- It is crucial to know and comprehend the herbs we gather, including their life cycles, growing environments, and therapeutic effects. This information enables us to choose the best times and methods for harvesting and the right amounts to take. We ensure that we collect the plants sustainably and responsibly by continuously learning about and researching them.

- Sustainable herb-gathering methods entail taking herbs without endangering the long-term viability of plant populations or their natural environments. Some crucial techniques include:
  - **Harvesting selectively**: Don't take all the plants in one location; only take what you need. So that it can recover and live on, leaving a sizable chunk of the people alone.
  - **Harvesting with care**: Avoid harm to the surrounding plants and their habitats when harvesting. Use clean, sharp equipment to produce clean cuts and minimize needless damage.
  - **Monitoring growth is essential**: To prevent over-harvesting, consider the plant's growth rate, state of conservation, and degree of sensitivity. Harvesting rare, threatened, or extinction-risked plants should be avoided.
  - **Taking only what is extra**: It's best to gather herbs where they are plenty rather than depleting populations in short supply. Harvest from regions where the plants are flourishing and have an abundance to sustain their reproduction ability.
- One of the most crucial principles is respecting ecosystems and biodiversity. When picking herbs, sustainable practices consider the greater ecosystem and biodiversity in addition to the individual plants. Think about how your collection will affect other species, including those that depend on the herb for survival, such as insects, animals, and other plants. While picking herbs, do not harm or destroy other plants or habitats.
- It is highly significant for having legal and ethical considerations. It is essential to abide by all applicable state, local, and federal laws and regulations regarding the collection of herbs. Recognize and respect any limitations on harvesting, such as protected areas or required permissions. Additionally, be conscious of any indigenous or cultural rights connected to the flora and seek the necessary partnerships or approvals from local communities.
- One should support regional economies and sustainable trade. Take sustainability's social and economic facets into account when sourcing herbs. Support regional herb producers and gatherers who use ecological and ethical practices wherever possible. This promotes fair commerce, boosts regional economies, and safeguards conventional knowledge.
- Those engaging in ethical and sustainable herb collection should seek to adopt regenerative practices beyond simple sustainability. This entails enhancing the well-being and vitality of the ecosystems and plants we interact with. Planting native plants, maintaining medicinal herb gardens, or assisting with habitat restoration projects are a few examples of regenerative practices.
- Collaboration and knowledge exchange is another significant principle. Knowledge exchange throughout the community is essential for sustainable and ethical herb collection. We can always learn from each other's experiences, knowledge, and experience to advance our practices. This can be accomplished through seminars, conventions, internet discussion boards, or collaborations with neighborhood groups and educational institutions.
- Learning the principles of sustainable and ethical herb collection entails methods that protect the long-term well-being of ecosystems and plants while showing respect for the populations and cultures involved. We can only reap the rewards of herbs while preserving and enhancing the natural world by adhering to these fundamental principles.
- Planting herbs even without the medicinal purpose is beneficial. Most herbs purify the air quality and keep a lot of viruses contained through air at a distance from its surroundings.

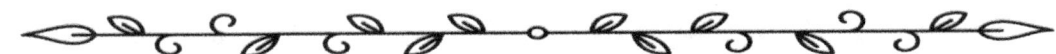

Practical Tips for Sustainable and Ethical Herb Gathering

Here are some recommendations and tips for picking herbs sustainably and ethically:

- **Learn and do your homework:** Before beginning your herb picking, familiarize yourself with the plants you intend to gather. Find all about their identity, growth patterns, and therapeutic qualities. Examine the state of their conservation and any rules or limitations affecting their harvest.

- **Always seek permission:** Always ask permission from landowners or authorities before picking herbs on private or protected grounds to show respect for private property. Observe any warnings or restrictions on collecting herbs that have been displayed.

- **Harvest with awareness:** When gathering herbs, pick only what you need and ensure enough plants are left for future development and reproduction. Leaving a sizable section of the plants unharvested can prevent over-harvesting. Additionally, ensure that there is an excess of herbs to aid in plant regeneration by harvesting in herb-rich areas.

- **Utilize sustainable techniques and tools:** To reduce harm to the plants, use cutting implements that are clean and sharp. Avoid applying chemical pesticides or herbicides that could damage the area's plant, soil, or environment. If necessary, choose manual eradication or organic pest management techniques.

- **Maintain the integrity of the surrounding plants and ecosystems:** When picking herbs, do not harm the nearby plants, soil, or habitats. Steers clear of trampling delicate ecosystems or other plants. Additionally, be aware of any animal or insect habitats or nesting sites and do not disturb them.

- **Protect biodiversity:** Avoid collecting rare, threatened, or endangered plant species to help safeguard biodiversity. Instead, gather common, plentiful herbs to maintain the ecosystem's balance.

- **Regenerative techniques:** Use regenerative techniques whenever possible to improve the health of the environment and the plants. This could entail participating in habitat restoration programs, growing medical herb gardens, or planting native herbs.

- **Create a journal and post your experiences:** Record your herb collection activities, noting the places, amounts, and techniques employed. By keeping a record of your procedures, you may reflect on them and make improvements. You'll also be able to impart important information to those who are enthusiastic about sustainable herb collection.

- **Respect for Different Traditions:** When picking herbs that cultural or indigenous people customarily utilize, you should respect their traditions and knowledge. Ensure you are not appropriating or taking advantage of their cultural history by asking for their advice, cooperation, or permission.

- **Fair-trade and local community support:** When buying or obtaining herbs, use fair-trade products that assist local communities and employ sustainable harvesting methods. Consider purchasing from regional farmers, herbalists, or groups dedicated to ethical and sustainable herb collection.

- We may contribute to preserving plant populations, ecosystems, and cultural legacy while ethically reaping the benefits of herbs by following this useful advice and recommendations for sustainable and ethical herb collection.

When discussing the tips for sustainable and ethical herb gathering, how can we neglect the significance of learning useful tips such as when and how to harvest different types of herbs? There are many things to consider when harvesting different kinds of herbs, including the plant species, the portions of the plant to be gathered, and the intended application (medical, culinary, or other). Following fundamental principles should be followed:

- **Harvesting at the right time:** It is essential for enhancing the flavor and potency of herbs. Herbs should be harvested at their prime, before or during blossoming. Their active ingredients and essential oils are at their peak concentration. On the other hand, certain herbs are better gathered after flowering and others before. Investigate specific plants to learn when to use each herb.
- **Harvesting leaves and flowers:** The leaves and flowers are the main components of most culinary and medicinal herbs. Be careful not to harm the main stem when collecting these bits severely. Use sharp, properly clean scissors or pruning shears to make clean cuts above a node or leaf junction. Basil, mint, and parsley are a few examples of plants whose outer leaves can be harvested while the inner leaves are left to continue growing.
- **Harvesting roots:** Some herbs, like ginseng, dandelion, and Valerian, are prized for their roots. Use a shovel to dig around the plant to gather the roots carefully. Gently shake off any extra soil and cut off any shriveled or damaged areas. Before continuing, give the roots a quick rinse with water and give them a thorough drying.
- **Harvesting seeds:** It's important to wait until the seeds are fully developed and dry on the plant before gathering herbs for their seeds. Cut the seed heads or pods off at the base using a pair of precise pruners or scissors to collect them. The seed heads should be put in a clean paper bag or other container to dry entirely. When the seed heads are dry, gently rub or crush them to release the seeds.
- **Herbs must be dried:** They must be properly dried after being harvested to maintain their quality and shelf life. Small bundles of stems should be hung upside down in a warm, well-ventilated area away from the sun. Alternatively, arrange the roots, blossoms, or leaves on a dry rack or clean screen. Stir or turn them frequently to guarantee equal drying and ward off mold or mildew.
- **Proper herbs storage:** Herbs should be stored appropriately after drying to maintain their effectiveness and avoid moisture or insect infestation. Keep dried herbs away from direct sunshine, heat, and humidity in tidy, sealed jars or containers. To maintain track of freshness, write the name and harvest date on the label of each jar. Herbs should always be kept in a cool, dark pantry or cabinet.
- **Consider the plant's life cycle:** Certain herbs are biennial or annual, while others are perennial. Different harvesting methods are necessary for perennial herbs to maintain long-term health and vigor. Perennial plants should not have all their leaves harvested, especially in the first year, to give them time to develop sturdy roots and last the winter.

For guidance on the plants, you desire to harvest, visit reliable herbal publications and resources, or speak with knowledgeable herbalists or gardeners. The quality, flavor, and medicinal qualities of the herbs you pick will be enhanced if you customize your harvesting methods for each herb.

The Role of Community in Sustainable Herb Gathering

Involving the community, educating the public, and encouraging sustainable herb-gathering practices are essential. We can all work together to maintain plant populations, preserve ecosystems, and promote a greater regard for nature by involving the community and spreading the word about how important sustainability is.

Community participation promotes cooperation, knowledge exchange, and experience sharing among herb gatherers, growers, indigenous communities, and locals. This makes it possible to disseminate best practices, conventional wisdom, and fresh research results that support sustainable herb collection methods. The involvement of the community can also aid in identifying and addressing any negative effects or difficulties linked to herb collection, enabling the creation of suitable solutions and regulations.

Education is essential for fostering sustainable herb collecting because it equips people with the knowledge and skills, they need to make wise decisions. Workshops, seminars, and training courses covering plant identification, growth

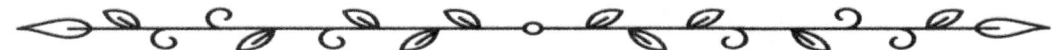

cycles, harvesting methods, and the value of conservation are examples of educational endeavors. By arming people with this information, they may actively aid in preserving herbs and their natural habitats while comprehending ethical behavior's value.

Overall, participation in the community and educational opportunities promote a sense of care and accountability for our natural resources. Together, we can ensure that herbs will always be available while protecting the environments that enable their cultivation.

Summary

In a nutshell, the chapter Sustainability and Ethical Herb Gathering consists of the following key points:

- This chapter strongly emphasizes respectfully and responsibly gathering herbs for religious, gastronomic, and therapeutic uses.
- Some fundamental concepts include respect for the plants, knowledge, and comprehension of the herbs, sustainable harvesting methods, observance of ethical and legal obligations, assistance for local people, and sustainable trading.
- Additional ideas emphasize knowledge exchange, collaboration, plant partnership, and regenerative practices.
- Learning and studying, getting permission, harvesting mindfully, maintaining the integrity of plants and habitats, protecting biodiversity, implementing regenerative practices, documenting and sharing experiences, respecting cultural practices, and aiding local communities are some useful advice.
- Community involvement and education are crucial to encourage sustainable herb harvesting, as they foster cooperation, information sharing, responsible behavior, and stewardship towards nature.

Growing your Own Herb Garden:
a Step-by-Step Guide

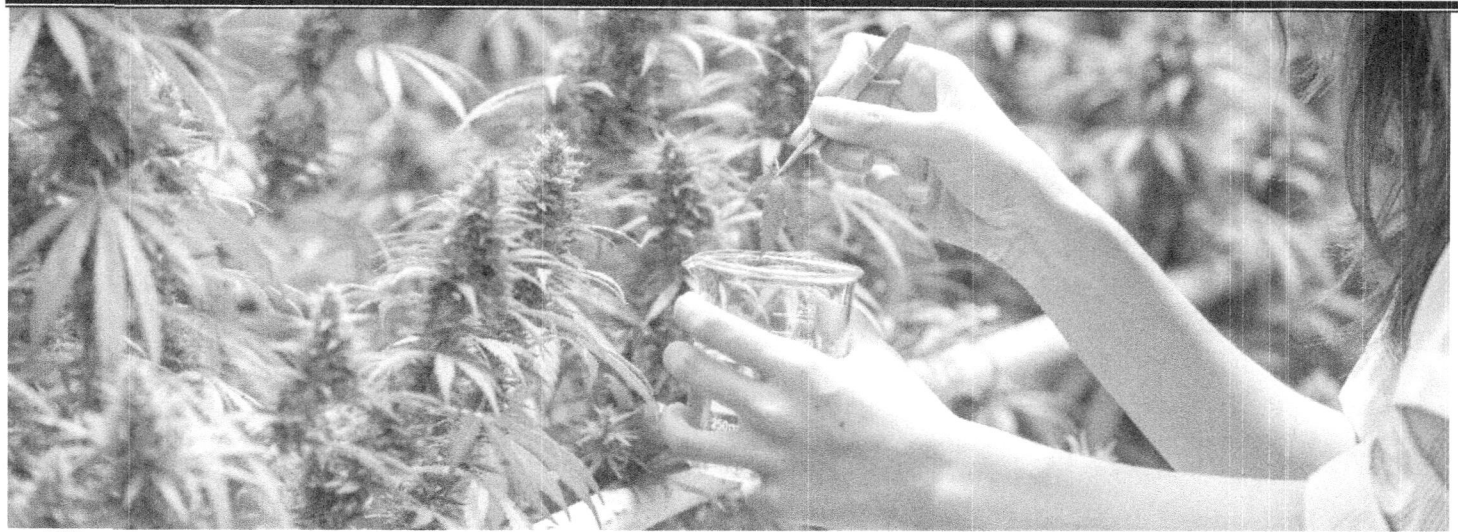

Creating your own herbal garden is a fun and satisfying endeavor that enables you to always have a supply of fresh, fragrant herbs close at hand. Whether you have a large backyard or a tiny balcony, cultivating an herbal garden is a wonderful way to get closer to nature, improve your cooking, and learn more about herbal cures. We'll lead you through starting your own herbal garden in this tutorial, from choosing the perfect herbs to ensuring they get the proper care and upkeep.

This guide will provide the information and inspiration you need to build a flourishing and plentiful herbal garden that will enrich your life for years to come, whether you are an experienced gardener or are just getting started. Let's begin this wonderful journey of creating and caring for your herbal retreat.

The Benefits of Growing Your Own Home Garden

Beyond having access to fresh vegetables, having a garden at home offers many advantages. You can enjoy the splendor of nature and the numerous benefits of taking care of your garden while living a more sustainable, independent, and joyful lifestyle. The following are some of the main benefits of maintaining your garden:

Access to tasty and fresh produce: Compared to store-bought alternatives, homegrown fruits, vegetables, and herbs offer unrivaled freshness and flavor. You can select and grow the types that best suit your palate, resulting in lively, nutrient-rich, and tasty produce.

- **Saving money:** Having your garden can save you money over time. Although the initial cost of seeds, soil, and gardening equipment may seem excessive, the continuous expense of routinely buying produce can be far greater. Your herbal garden can make you save money by growing your food and reducing reliance on store-bought produce.
- **Better nutrition and health:** Since you control the soil's quality, pesticide use, and harvest time, homegrown produce is frequently more nutrient-dense. Since you have instant access to newly harvested veggies and herbs, you may consume them when they are at their nutritional peak, which is good for your general health and well-being.

- **More security for home:** An additional layer of security is offered by having a home garden during catastrophes or unforeseen circumstances, such as natural disasters or disruptions in the food supply chains. Feeding your family and yourself with the food you raise yourself can be quite useful in times of need.

- **An outside area that is aesthetically pleasing:** Home gardens make your outside area look better and provide peace and beauty to the area. You can experience a warm and unwinding environment all year long thanks to the vivid colors, enticing scents, and lush foliage.

- **Sustainability in the environment:** Growing a garden at home encourages sustainability and lessens your ecological imprint. Growing your own food eliminates the need for packing, shipping, and the overuse of pesticides and herbicides frequently connected to industrial agriculture practices.

- **Stress reduction and mental health:** It has been established that gardening is a therapeutic activity that lowers stress, anxiety, and depression. It re-establishes your connection to nature, gives you a sense of accomplishment, and fosters a serene atmosphere conducive to relaxation.

- **A beneficial educational experience:** Gardening may be a beneficial educational experience for both adults and children. It provides a chance to comprehend the plant life cycle, recognize the value of nature, instill responsibility, and promote a sense of independence.

- **Increased exercise:** Gardening involves physical energy to plant, dig, weed, and harvest. Regular participation in these activities increases physical activity levels, fostering a healthier lifestyle and better fitness.

- **Diversity of plants and animals:** small animals like birds, bees, butterflies, and helpful insects can live in home gardens. You help preserve regional biodiversity by fostering a warm atmosphere with various plants and flowers in a garden.

Starting a home garden offers various advantages beyond just the vegetables you plant, whether you have a large backyard or little pot room. It offers a satisfying and enlightening experience that feeds your body and soul.

Choosing the Right Herbs for Your Garden

A successful and pleasant gardening experience depends on selecting the appropriate herbs for your garden. You can create a diversified collection of herbs that will flourish in your garden and satisfy your culinary and medicinal demands by considering personal preferences, climatic suitability, and maintenance requirements.

When selecting the herbs for your garden, it's important to consider your preferences, intended purpose, temperature, and available growing space. The following advice will assist you in making wise decisions:

- **Considering your preferences:** Consider your unique preferences for flavors and smells as a starting point. Note the herbs frequently used in the foods you appreciate or like to add to your cooking. By doing this, you can be confident that your selected herbs will improve your culinary endeavor's.

- **Determine your goals:** Identify your goals and intended usage for the herbs before using them. Are you primarily interested in using herbs for cooking, brewing tea, creating cures, or just for their pleasant aroma? Choose herbs that are compatible with the usage you have in mind because they all serve different functions.

- **Climate suitability:** Verify the hardiness zones and local climate characteristics. While certain plants thrive in favorable environments, others are more tolerant of colder or hotter climes. Pick herbs suited to your area's climate to ensure their survival and ideal growth.

- **Determine the size of your garden:** Determine the size of the space you have for your herb garden. You can consider planting various herbs in your garden if it is spacious. Instead, choose small or dwarf kinds that may be planted in pots or vertical gardens if you are short on space. To prevent overpopulation and resource competition, make the appropriate plans and allow for adequate spacing.

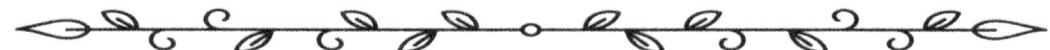

- **Sunlight needs:** Consider how much sunlight your garden gets throughout the day. Most herbs need at least six hours of direct sunlight for optimum growth. Pick herbs that work with the lighting in your garden. Mint and parsley work well in shady regions, whereas rosemary and thyme flourish in direct sunlight.

- **Right efforts and care:** Consider how much effort and care you will put into maintenance and care. While certain herbs, like ore consider your soil's condition and composition when determining its needs. While some herbs require sandy or damp soil, others do best in well-drained soil. To produce the optimum growth circumstances for your chosen herbs, consider any modifications or adjustments that may be required.

- **Knowledge of water needs:** Consider the water needs of various herbs while determining your tolerance to drought. Pick drought-tolerant herbs like lavender or thyme if you live in a dry climate or like low-maintenance plants. These plants are more resilient to arid environments.

- **Sensitivity of herbs:** Find out which herbs are resistant to pests and diseases by researching their susceptibility. While some herbs, like basil or cilantro, may need extra protection or vigilance against typical garden pests, others, like sage or rosemary, have natural pest-repellent capabilities. Choose herbs that are reputed to be hardy and less susceptible to pests and diseases in your region.

- **Right Research:** Research on companion planting to increase the productivity and health of your garden. Some herbs interact well with other plants, preventing pests and promoting development. For instance, growing basil close to tomatoes can help keep pests away and enhance their flavor.

- **Knowledge about different growth patterns:** Discover each herb's growth patterns, including spreading, clumping, and trailing. Think about how the herbs will develop and whether they will work well with other plants in your garden.

- **Beautify your herbal garden:** Consider including herbs with edible flowers, such as chamomile or nasturtium, to add visual appeal and improve your culinary creations. Edible flowers also have ornamental value. Some herbs, like lavender or lemon balm, can make excellent garden ornaments because of their lovely foliage and aromatic properties.

When choosing your herbs, remember these characteristics to help you design a successful and beautiful herbal garden. Enjoy selecting herbs that suit your tastes, preferences, and growing circumstances because gardening will be more pleasurable and rewarding. The long-term goal is to keep fresh and stored herbs at all times in order to fight off basic diseases and even to just enjoy the multiple benefits that nature brings to our doorstep.

Planning Your Herbal Garden

Planning your herbal garden is the first exciting and important step to a successful garden. You can create a garden that meets your requirements by carefully considering elements, including area, objectives, herb selection, and maintenance needs.

The planning step entails determining the available space, learning about the requirements of the herbs you want to grow, creating the layout, and setting up care and maintenance. You may make a lovely and fruitful herbal garden with a well-thought-out plan that gives you fresh, flavorful herbs for culinary and medicinal uses.

Planning for your herbal garden is the vital first step that lays the groundwork for a prosperous and profitable garden. You may create a garden that matches your needs, makes the most of your available space and resources, and guarantees a plentiful harvest using a systematic approach. Following are some step-by-step instructions that will assist you in planning your herbal garden:

- **Examine your area:** Establish the size of the space you have for your herb garden. Think about indoor areas with enough natural light and outside possibilities like a backyard, balcony, or windowsill. Take measurements

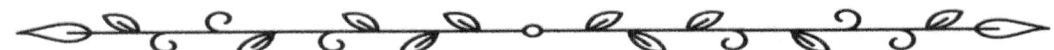

and account for any architectural or environmental elements that may impact the garden, such as wind exposure or building shade.

- **Set your objectives:** Gain knowledge about the herbs: Learn about the requirements of the herbs you want to grow by researching their needs. Consider the demand for sunlight, preferred soil, water needs, spacing, and potential companion planting. You can select herbs that are suitable for your area and the circumstances in your garden with the aid of this research.

- **Creating the layout:** Plan the general layout of your garden area and the locations of each herb. Arrange the herbs considering their size and growth patterns. Group herbs with comparable water and light requirements together for the convenience of management. Allow room to access each plant to water, harvest, and maintain it.

- **Choose your planting techniques:** Consider growing herbs in containers, raised beds, or the open ground. Every technique offers advantages and things to keep in mind. Containers or raised beds can be useful and adaptable in smaller settings.

- **Choose the right season:** Consider which herbs are biennials, perennials, or annuals when planning for seasonal fluctuations. Plan for herbs that may die in the winter or require protection during the colder months by considering the shifting seasons. Your herbal garden will remain healthy and productive for a long time if you do this.

- **Plan the list of Supplies:** Make a list of the supplies you'll need, like soil, compost, containers, tools, and supports, and then go out and gather them. For planting, watering, and pruning your herbs, ensure access to good soil and the right tools.

- **Establish a schedule:** Plan when to plant, transplant, and harvest your herbs. Please consider their growth rates, the length of time till maturity, and any unique care needs. This calendar will keep you organized and guarantee that the herbs are properly cared for throughout the year.

- **Start small and grow:** If you're new to gardening, think about starting with a small garden of herbs and gradually increasing it as you acquire expertise and confidence. This strategy enables you to concentrate on a manageable number of plants and guarantee their healthy development.

The process of planning your own herbal garden is an exciting adventure, but at the same time, it requires a lot of hard work, research, and planning and is a long-term process. In addition to giving, you a plentiful supply of fragrant and savory herbs, a well-designed herbal garden allows you to connect with nature, benefiting your culinary and medical endeavours. Making remedies for multiple uses will be easy and almost free. Having access to nature's gifts have an amazing effect on your body even by looking at the green, purple, and multi-coloured plants.

Remember that planning your herbal garden is a continuous process; adjustments may be required as your garden changes. You'll be ready to design a lovely and fruitful herbal garden if you carefully analyze your area, objectives, and herb needs. All the above guidelines will help you achieve a gorgeous herbal garden but follow all the guidelines to achieve your desired results.

Planting and Caring for Your Herbs: A Step-by-Step Process

Herbs have proven their worth in the medicinal industry. Apart from getting ready-made medicines from a professional for each thing, it would be a lot easier to always get some basic herbs in your garden and at your disposal.

According to Ayurveda and Chinese medicine, some natural remedies can be made with pre-available ingredients, like; garlic, honey, onion, cumin seed, cinnamon stick, etc. But still there are a lot more herbs that can benefit your everyday life and make your immunity stronger by using them. Before having an herb garden at your home, you need to be sure

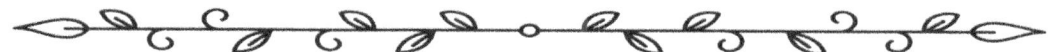

that you are fully equipped with the right tools and gadgets to embark on the journey of natural healing from your home garden. You will need to be sure you have the following things before you start your herb garden:

- **Tools for gardening:** Like every sort of gardening and harvesting, it is important to have the tools. You will need pots for planting the seeds or roots, shovel, scraper, right quality of soil, etc.
- **Proper area:** In your home you need to have a proper area for growing herbs. Each herb may require different amount of sunshine, water, etc. You need to be able to provide direct sunlight to many herbs each day for the herbs to bloom fully. Make sure if you don't have a proper garden, you put the plants near a window that receives direct sunlight.
- **Be aware of your local climate and plant herbs accordingly:** Not all herbs can survive in extreme cold weather of Canada or the Poles, so if you are from those regions, you will not be able to harvest garlic, lemon, etc. Before buying seeds or roots of herbs, you need to make sure the climate of your city, is growth-friendly for the herbs you plan on having in your garden.

You can grow many herbs in your garden and here is how you can do it.

Step 1: Choosing Your Herbs

First, you need to decide what types of herbs you want to grow. Consider what you use most in your kitchen, the amount of space you have, and the climate of your region. Some common herbs include basil, parsley, rosemary, thyme, oregano, and mint. There are also many other herbs which would need a slightly larger area. If you have a proper garden dedicated to herbs, you can easily plant those herbs like; turmeric roots, lemon, etc.

Step 2: Purchasing and Planting Your Herbs

Purchase your herbs from a local nursery or garden center. Herbs can be grown from seeds, but for beginners, it's often easier to start with established plants. You can buy an already sprouted and potted plant from a local nursery and start from there.

- Prepare the garden soil by removing weeds and adding compost or other organic matter to improve the nutrient content.
- Dig a hole that is twice as wide and just as deep as the root ball of your herb plant.
- Place the herb in the hole, ensuring the top of the root ball is level with the soil surface.
- Backfill the hole with soil, gently firming it around the base of the plant. At all steps, be extremely gentle with the roots of the herbs, you don't want to damage the roots or effects its growth in any negative manner.

Step 3: Watering Your Herbs

- Water the herbs immediately after planting to settle the soil.
- Water them regularly but avoid over-watering as most herbs prefer soil that's slightly dry to the touch.

Step 4: Fertilizing Your Herbs

- Apply a balanced organic fertilizer to your herbs about once a month during the growing season. This will provide them with the nutrients they need to grow and produce flavorful leaves.
- Make sure the fertilizer is good enough to be used on the herbs and is not damaging to the roots.

Step 5: Managing Pests and Diseases

Herbs are generally low-maintenance plants, but they can still be affected by pests and diseases.

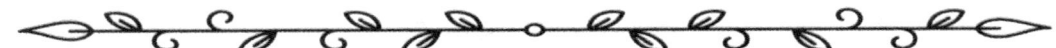

- Inspect your herbs regularly for signs of pests or disease, such as discolored leaves or unusual spots.
- If you find pests, try to identify them and use the appropriate organic pest control method. This could involve manually removing pests, using natural predators, or applying an organic pesticide. Do your research before taking any measures so that the plant doesn't get damaged further.
- If a plant appears diseased, remove the affected parts immediately to prevent the disease from spreading.

Step 6: Pruning and Harvesting

- Regularly pruning your herbs will encourage bushier growth. For most herbs, you can simply pinch off the tops of the plants with your fingers.
- Harvest herbs by cutting off stems with sharp, clean scissors. It's best to harvest in the morning after the dew has dried but before the sun gets too hot.

Planting and gardening are fun if you enjoy it. Be sure to follow all the preventative measures and take proper care of your herbs to make them beneficial for you to its maximum capacity.

Harvesting and Storing Herbs

Harvesting any plant needs to be done with care and love. Plants are living being and need proper care at each step of the process. Same is the case with herbs, like, giving proper water, sunlight, having a good quality soil, is important, harvesting it is equally important.

There is an entire process that needs to be done to harvest the herbs and the make it ready to be stored properly to be used in different things. Most likely, the herbs that you harvest will not all be used all at once, so you will have to store the herb in a correct manner to preserve its benefits for a longer period.

Harvesting Herbs

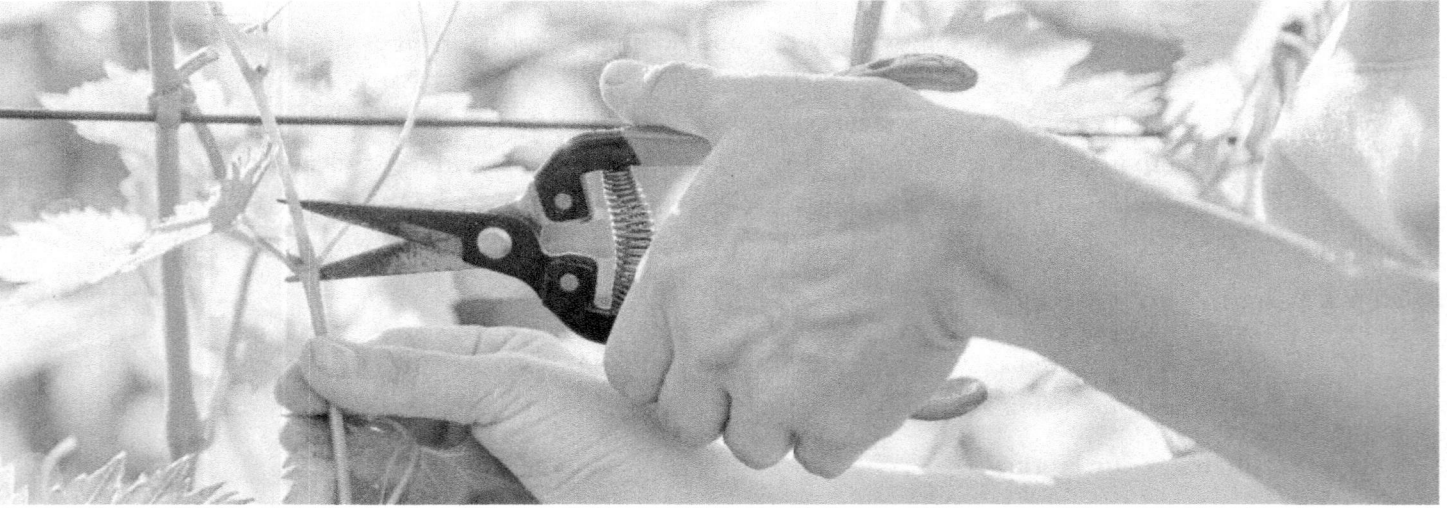

Each step of harvesting needs to be done, timing is a matter of crucial importance. If you do not harvest an herb or a plant at the right time, you might not be able to get most of its vital chemicals that you require.

- **Time of Harvesting**: Herbs should typically be harvested just before the flowers bloom for the best flavor. The best time of day to harvest herbs is early morning, after the dew has dried but before the sun gets too hot. The heat of the sun tends to wilt the plants and can reduce their oil content, which is where much of their

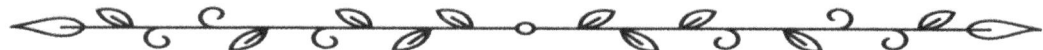

flavor comes from. Start early and before going ahead and cutting the herb make sure you are doing it in the right way.

- **Cutting the Herbs**: Using a sharp pair of scissors or pruning shears, cut off the herbs, being careful not to damage the plant. Aim to cut just above a set of growing leaves. This will encourage the plant to branch out and grow more foliage. Not all the plant should be ripped out, be gentle and take only what you need, if taking for immediate use. Do not waste those magic stems and leaves.

- **Gathering the Herbs**: Gather up your herbs but be gentle - you don't want to bruise the leaves. Each herb has a part that is needed, not the entire plant. So just take that part and let the other parts of plant be undisturbed and undamaged.

- **Cleaning**: Rinse the herbs gently under cold water to remove any soil or bugs, then pat them dry with paper towels or let them air dry. Make sure they are completely dry before storing them to prevent Mold and rot. This is for all types of plants and fruits generally. Any kind of moisture can damage the harvested product.

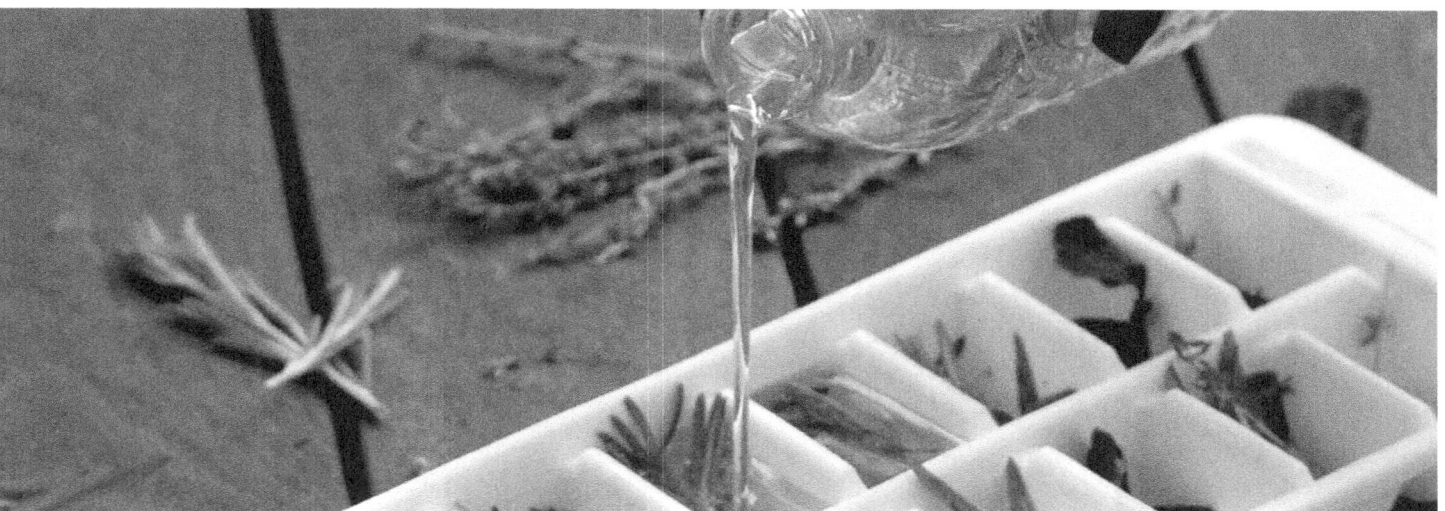

Storing Herbs

After harvesting comes the important and final step, the one that you did all this hard work for, storing the herbs to be used.

- **Refrigeration**: For short-term storage, place fresh herbs in an unsealed plastic bag in the crisper drawer of your refrigerator. Some herbs, like parsley and cilantro, can also be stored upright in a glass of water with a loose plastic bag over the top, like cut flowers. This is the easiest and most common practice for storing basic herbs that would be used in less than a week.

- **Freezing**: For long-term storage, herbs can be frozen. There are two popular methods for freezing herbs:

- **Whole leaf freezing**: Spread the herbs out on a baking sheet and freeze them. Once frozen, they can be transferred to a freezer-safe container or bag. This method works best with hardier herbs like rosemary and thyme. Freezing preserves the important nutrients of the herbs without letting the plant wilt.

- **Ice cube freezing**: Chop the herbs up and place them in an ice cube tray, then fill the tray with water or olive oil. Once frozen, these cubes can be dropped directly into soups or sauces. This is a good and hassle-free way for immediate use of the herbs. It is also a common practice in homemade skin care remedies.

- **Drying**: Herbs can also be dried for long-term storage. Tie the herbs in small bundles and hang them upside down in a warm, dry, well-ventilated place out of direct sunlight. Once completely dry, store them in airtight containers away from heat and light. Crumble them when you're ready to use them, like dried mint, parsley,

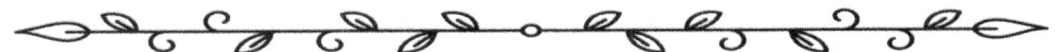

etc. You can use the dried herbs to even garnish your food or in the recipe of several dishes. Most Asian cuisines use a lot of herbs in its recipes.

Remember that dried herbs have a more concentrated flavor than fresh, so you will need to adjust the quantities when using them in recipes. A good rule of thumb is to use one-third to one-half as much dried herb as you would fresh.

When stored properly, the herbs and the herb garden is going to be of great value to your family in terms of cooking, treating ailments, and even supplementing your diet, making some interesting beauty hacks and many more diversified ways of use.

Summary

Growing your own herb garden is a lot less hard work compared to the benefits you will reap in almost no time. Most of the herbs are easy to grow and require very less care, like; mint, parsley, etc. Here is a brief rundown of what we covered in this chapter:

- Multiple benefits of growing your own herbs, you can have easier access to the herb at the time of need even if you had not harvested the plant yet. There are multiple benefits even from the ecosystem point, a home garden has health benefits apart from those which comes by using the herbs in a particular manner.
- It is important to choose the right herbs for your herb garden. Not every type of herb can grow in your local climate. Be careful while choosing what and which herb you will grow. You will have to be cautious about the soil type as not all soils are good for all herbs.
- If you do not have a garden or even within a garden, you need to dedicate a place for your herbs. Herbs may need direct sunlight, or fresh air exposure to bloom fully. Keep in mind the factors like; layout of the garden, the exact location where your herb plant can thrive, preparing the soil, etc.
- Planting and caring for your herbs are another major step. Some herbs are easy going and don't require much effort. But you need to be sure when to water, how to keep the soil to its maximum nutritional level, etc.
- When all is done, now is the time to enjoy the fruit of your hard work and patience. You can now harvest and store the herbs. Harvesting is a process that needs to be done with care, be gentle with the plant and make sure it is the right time for the plant to be harvested. Mostly, early morning is the most suitable time. You can store the herbs in many ways, choose what suits you the best, like; freezing, drying or just simply keeping it in the fridge to be used in a few days.

Top Herbal Antibiotics:
Detailed Profiles and Uses

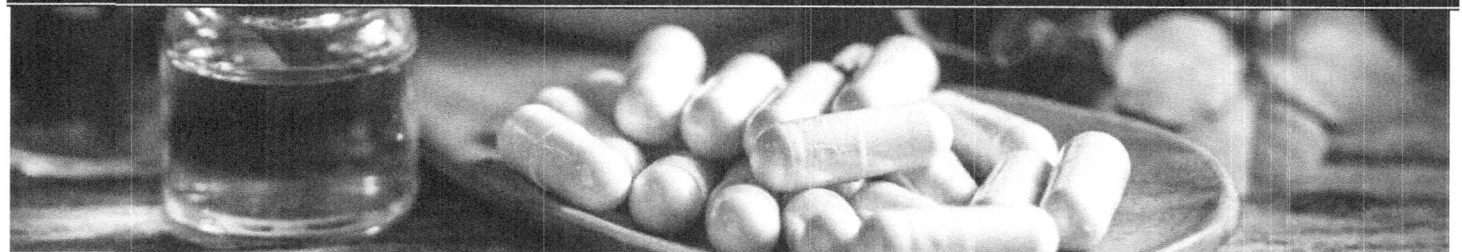

Introduction to Herbal Profiles

Before diving into individual herbal antibiotics, it's essential to understand the concept of herbal profiles. Herbal profile refers to comprehensive information about a particular herb, including its botanical name, historical uses, active compounds, proven benefits, recommended dosages, potential side effects, and any interactions with other medications. This profiling helps users and practitioners have a holistic view of the herb, ensuring safe and effective use.

Herbal antibiotics are naturally occurring substances extracted from plants that are known for their antibacterial properties. Unlike synthetic antibiotics, which are formulated in labs, herbal antibiotics have been used for centuries to treat various illnesses and conditions. This section delves deep into the concept of herbal antibiotics, their types, effectiveness, and how they can be incorporated into modern medical practices.

Types of Herbal Antibiotics

Herbal antibiotics can be broadly categorized into three types:
- **Broad-Spectrum Herbal Antibiotics:** These work against a wide range of bacteria and are often used as a general anti-infective. Examples include garlic, turmeric, and Echinacea.
- **Narrow-Spectrum Herbal Antibiotics:** These are effective against specific types of bacteria. For instance, golden-seal is generally effective against gram-positive bacteria.
- **Adjunctive Herbal Antibiotics:** These types of herbal medicines enhance the effectiveness of synthetic antibiotics when used in conjunction. They might help in reducing inflammation, boosting immunity, or aiding in digestion.

While there's ongoing research into the efficacy of herbal antibiotics, preliminary results suggest that some herbal extracts do exhibit strong antibacterial properties. It is essential to note that while herbal antibiotics can be effective, they are not a direct substitute for synthetic antibiotics in severe bacterial infections. It's essential to consult a healthcare provider before beginning any herbal regimen, especially for pregnant or breastfeeding women, children, or individuals with preexisting health conditions.

Herbal antibiotics fall under the category of dietary supplements in many countries, which means they are not subjected to the same rigorous testing as pharmaceutical drugs. This lack of regulation often makes it challenging to determine the potency, purity, and safety of these products.

In this chapter profiles, uses, precautions, side effects, and methods to grow each herbal plant is discussed in detail. Most of the plants discussed are easy to grow in a home garden and yield multiple health benefits.

Echinacea

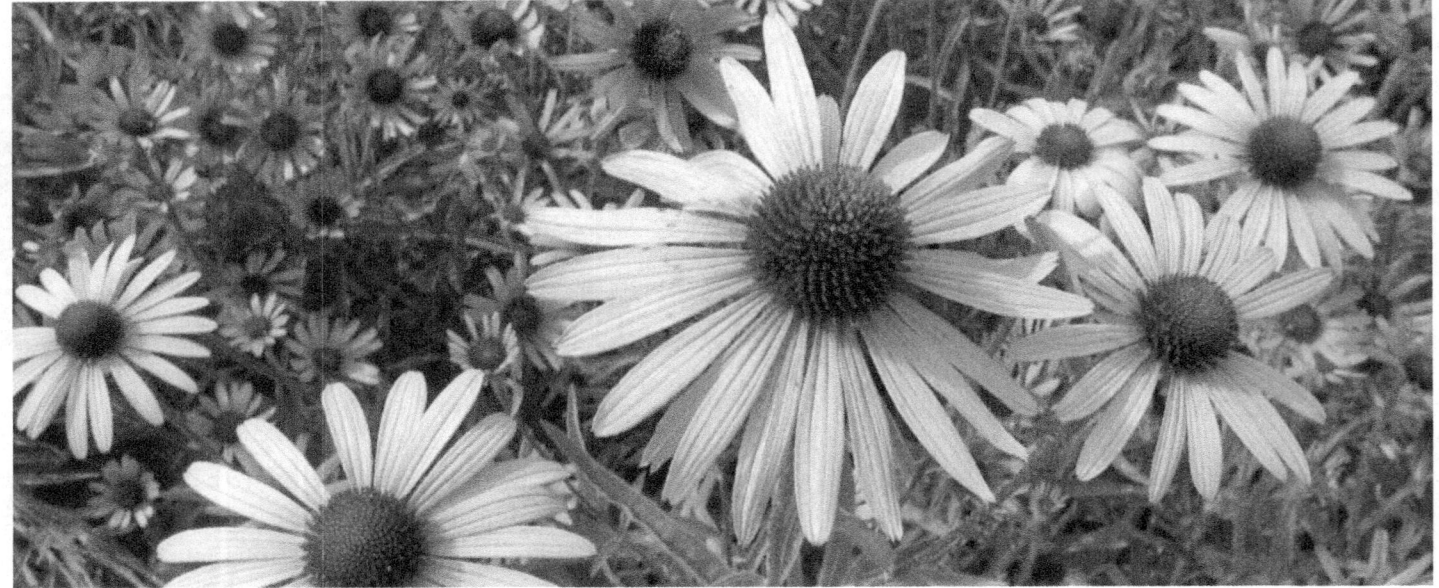

Echinacea is a plant with flowers ranging in various colors. It is found in moist, dry, open wooded prairies, mostly in eastern and central North America. It is commonly known as the coneflower. The flower plant was found effective for many internal issues including gut health.

Botanical Name: Echinacea purpurea (though there are other species like Echinacea angustifolia and Echinacea pallida)

Family: Asteraceae

Common Names: Purple coneflower, American coneflower

Uses as an Herbal Antibiotic:

Echinacea has been touted for its therapeutic properties for centuries, especially among indigenous communities in North America. The flower and its leaves are known for its healing properties. It is important to understand Echinacea's medicinal purpose in order to avail full benefits from it.

- **Immune System Boost:** Echinacea is a powerful herb, and it stimulates the immune system, making it beneficial for warding off colds and flu. It can be given in the form of tea by steeping it in hot water for a couple of minutes. This remedy has been tried and tested for ages.

- **Antiviral and Antibacterial:** It's not a direct replacement for antibiotics, echinacea has shown promise against several bacterial and viral infections. For minor diseases, where people do not like to take antibiotics, it has served as an alternative. It soothes the pain and relaxes the mind.

- **Wound Healing:** Echinacea has been used traditionally to treat boils, skin infections, and other external wounds, owing to its antimicrobial and anti-inflammatory properties. A paste is created by crushing the flower and its leaves, other herbs can also be added to increase the effectiveness, then this paste is applied to the affected area.

- **Respiratory Health:** It's often recommended for respiratory ailments like bronchitis, sinusitis, and common colds. It has properties to soothe the throat and the lungs, making it a potential medicine to treat multiple diseases.

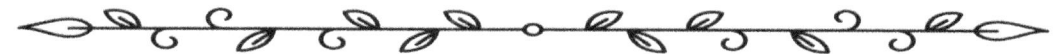

Precautions:

- **Allergies:** People allergic to plants in the Asteraceae family, such as ragweed, mums, marigolds, or daisies, might also be allergic to echinacea. A person aiming to treat an illness with Echinacea must first know if they are allergic to the herb or not.
- **Autoimmune Diseases:** Since echinacea stimulates the immune system, it might exacerbate symptoms of autoimmune disorders. It can cause discomfort and even activate a disease and cause pain and infections. It is better to not take this herb if one has an autoimmune disease.
- **Interactions:** It can interact with some medications, including those that suppress the immune system or affect the liver. Many medicines are not good to be taken together. Echinacea is a complex herb and cannot be taken with various other medicines, traditional or herbal.

Side Effects:

While echinacea is generally considered safe for most people, some might experience:
- Dizziness or headaches
- Nausea or stomach discomfort
- Skin rashes or itching
- Worsening of asthma symptoms

It's essential to discontinue use and consult a physician if severe reactions or side effects are observed.

How to Grow Echinacea:

Echinacea is not only therapeutic but also a beautiful addition to gardens.

- **Planting:** Choose a sunny spot with well-draining soil. While Echinacea purpurea is the most common garden variety, other species might have specific growth requirements.
- **Seed Germination:** Cold stratify the seeds by placing them in a wet paper towel inside a plastic bag in the fridge for about 30 days. After that, sow them 1/8 inch deep in the soil.
- **Watering:** Echinacea is drought-resistant once established, but young plants need regular watering.
- **Maintenance:** It requires minimal care. Deadheading spent flowers can encourage more blooms, but leaving some can provide seeds for birds.
- **Harvesting:** If you're growing echinacea for its medicinal properties, the roots are often used and are best harvested in the fall from 3-4-year-old plants.

Growing echinacea at home can provide easy access to this potent herb. Still, educating oneself and consulting with professionals before using it as a remedy is essential.

Garlic

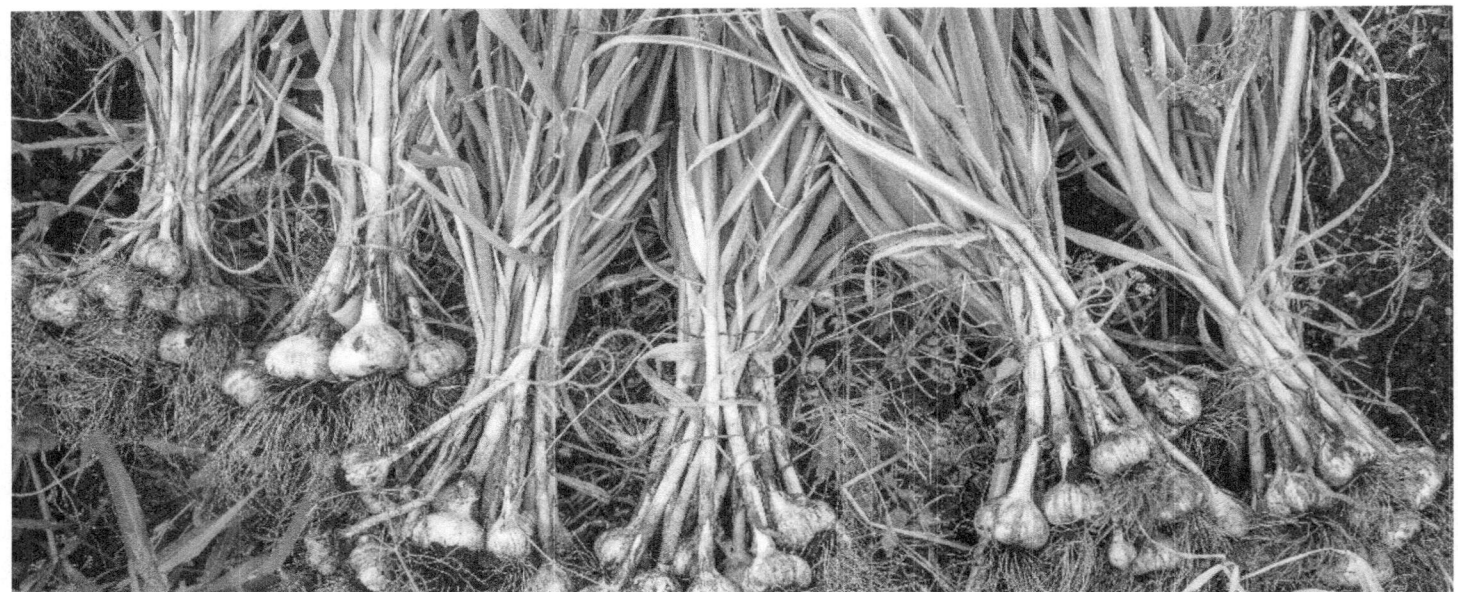

It is a versatile herb as it has been used since centuries to cure different health issues and even to make delicious cuisines. Garlic is easy to grow and is beneficial if you have it in your home, the smell may not be pleasant, but the other benefits outweigh the odor of this herb.

Botanical Name: Allium sativum

Family: Amaryllidaceae

Common Names: Garlic, Rocambole, Stinking Rose

Medicinal Properties:
Garlic has been celebrated for its myriad of health benefits and therapeutic properties, which include:
- **Anti-microbial:** Garlic contains allicin, a compound that has shown effectiveness against bacteria, fungi, parasites, and viruses. Garlic is used to treat infections and diseases internally and externally. Any fugal issue on the skin can be treated with the help of garlic mixed with few other herbs.
- **Cardiovascular Health:** Regular consumption of garlic is believed to improve heart health by reducing blood pressure, lowering cholesterol, and combating arteriosclerosis. It is also proven by traditional medicine that consumption of garlic is beneficial for cardiovascular health. Garlic also helps to keep the cholesterol levels under control.
- **Antioxidant:** Rich in antioxidants, garlic helps in neutralizing free radicals in the body, which can prevent cellular damage. Regular consumption of garlic, like in food, or making tea of garlic, helps with keeping the harmful cells neutralized.
- **Anti-inflammatory:** Some compounds in garlic have anti-inflammatory effects, which can help reduce inflammation in the body. Garlic absolves bloating and other gut issues keeping the metabolism in check.
- **Immune Boosting:** Garlic is known to enhance the body's immune cell function, potentially reducing the severity of colds and other mild illnesses. Garlic is a powerful healing agent of nature; it also has great benefits if you keep it near a kid who has flu or other immunity issues.

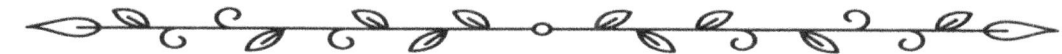

Uses as an Herbal Antibiotic:

- **Respiratory Infections:** Traditionally used for treating colds, bronchitis, and other respiratory infections.
- **Digestive Issues:** Garlic has been used to address various digestive ailments and is believed to combat certain harmful bacteria in the gut.
- **Skin Infections:** Applied topically, garlic can act against fungal skin infections like athlete's foot.
- **General Health:** Consuming garlic regularly can bolster the immune system, making the body more resilient against various pathogens.

Precautions:

- **Blood Thinners:** Garlic can act as a natural blood thinner, so it's essential to be cautious if you're already on blood-thinning medication. People suffering from cardiovascular issues are mostly on blood thinning medicines, it is advised to consult your health practitioner before taking garlic as an herbal antibiotic for any of your health issues.
- **Surgery:** Due to its blood-thinning properties, it's advisable to reduce garlic consumption before undergoing surgery. Garlic can thin the blood which can cause severe blood loss during the surgery. It is advised to stop consuming garlic as a medicine at least a week before your surgery is scheduled.
- **Digestive Issues:** Excessive consumption can lead to gastrointestinal issues in some individuals. Garlic is a strong herb, it has a strong aroma as well as a strong taste, some people may have issue in digesting garlic.

Side Effects:

- Garlic has a strong aroma; it can cause bad breath and body odor.
- Heartburn, gas, nausea, especially when consumed in large amounts.
- Skin irritation when applied topically as it is potentially strong and has some strong chemical that become active when garlic is crushed and applied.
- Reduced platelet aggregation, which can lead to increased bleeding. Garlic can make blood thinner, so it is not recommended to take it for medicinal use if a person is an easy bleeder.

How to Grow Garlic:

Growing garlic at home is relatively straightforward and rewarding.

- **Planting:** Garlic is usually planted in the fall. Break up garlic bulbs into individual cloves and plant them, pointy end up, about 2 inches deep and 4 inches apart.
- **Soil and Sun:** Garlic prefers full sun and fertile, well-draining soil.
- **Watering:** Keep the soil moist but not waterlogged. Once the foliage starts to turn yellow in late spring or early summer, reduce watering.
- **Harvesting:** When about half of the foliage turns yellow (usually in late spring or early summer), it's time to harvest. Gently dig around the bulbs and pull them out.
- **Curing:** After harvesting, let the garlic bulbs dry in a warm, dry place, out of direct sunlight for about a week. This curing process improves their storage capacity.

Remember, while garlic offers many health benefits, it's not a cure-all. Always consult with a healthcare professional when considering it for medicinal purposes.

Ginger

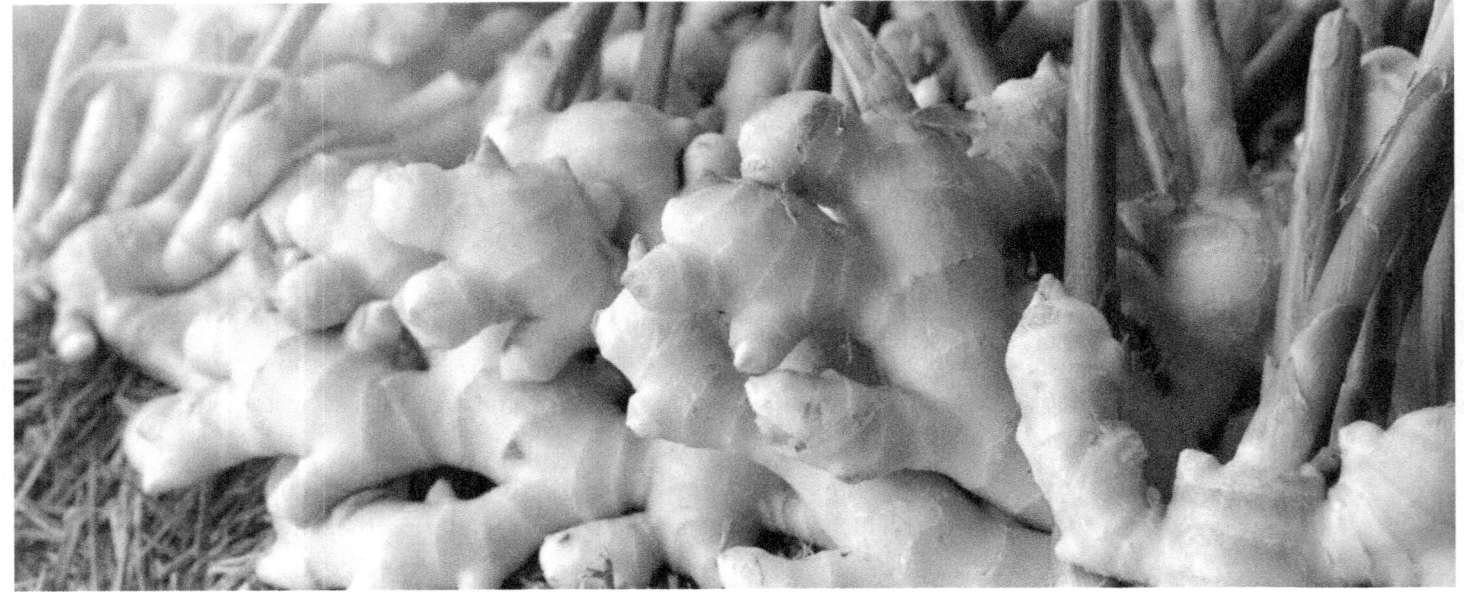

Ginger is a spicy herb, also used in most of the Asian cuisines. It is known to have multiple health benefits especially for women.

Botanical Name: Zingiber officinale

Family: Zingiberaceae

Common Names: Ginger root, Garden ginger

Medicinal Properties:

Ginger, with its spicy flavor and aromatic scent, has long been recognized for its range of medicinal attributes. It has proven to be a human friendly herb and can provide quick home remedies for a lot of issues faced on a regular basis. People of all age groups can benefit from its usage.

- **Anti-inflammatory:** Ginger contains gingerol, which has potent anti-inflammatory effects, making it beneficial for conditions such as arthritis. It relaxes the muscles and reduces the inflammation on joints.
- **Digestive Aid:** It's renowned for its ability to alleviate gastrointestinal irritation, stimulate saliva, and suppress gastric contractions as food and fluids move through the GI tract. A tea made with ginger is effective for increasing metabolism and clearing mucus from the windpipe, all in one go.
- **Anti-nausea:** Ginger is effective in preventing nausea, especially motion sickness, morning sickness during pregnancy, and chemotherapy-induced nausea. Ginger doesn't have negative effects if consumed by a pregnant lady, so it can be consumed to treat nausea, body aches and even sneezing issues.
- **Antioxidant:** The herb is rich in antioxidants, which combat free radicals in the body, thus reducing oxidative stress. It helps the body detoxify and release all the bad cells and toxins through the proper channels.
- **Analgesic:** Ginger may have pain-reducing properties, especially for menstrual pain. It is also a helpful herb when a person is suffering from poly-cystic ovary syndrome (PCOs)

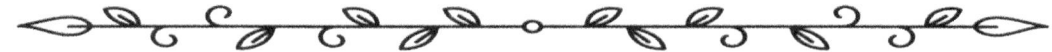

Uses as an Herbal Antibiotic:

- **Respiratory Tract Infections:** Ginger is used in many traditional remedies for treating respiratory infections and symptoms of the flu and common cold. It liquefies the mucus and helps the body get rid of it.
- **Mouth Bacteria:** The herb can act against oral bacteria linked to inflammatory diseases in the gums, such as gingivitis and periodontitis. Those who suffer from bleeding gums can increase intake of ginger in order to stop the gums from bleeding.
- **Digestive Tract Infections:** Gingerol can help in fighting harmful bacteria in the digestive tract. It aids the digestive process, making the metabolism faster. People who want to lose weight can also increase intake of ginger for healthier, cleaner internal organs.
- **Fungal Infections:** Ginger has shown potential in combating fungal infections. It can treat infections internally as well as topically.

Precautions:

- **Blood Thinning:** Ginger might slow blood clotting and should be used with caution by individuals on anticoagulant medications. Those who are already on blood thinning medication, may not want to use ginger or overuse it.
- **Gallstones:** Those with gallstones should consult a doctor before consuming more significant amounts, as it might increase bile flow causing more stones.
- **Pregnancy:** While ginger can help with morning sickness, excessive amounts should be avoided during pregnancy. As it can create acidity issues.

Side Effects:

- Heartburn
- Diarrhea
- Stomach discomfort
- Mouth or throat irritation, when consumed in large amounts

How to Grow Ginger:

Ginger is a tropical plant but can be grown indoors or in a greenhouse in colder climates. It needs proper care and cannot thrive in tough climates.

- **Starting:** Purchase fresh ginger rhizomes (roots) from a garden store or organic grocery store. Soak them overnight in water.
- **Planting:** Choose a wide, shallow pot. Fill it with potting soil and plant the rhizomes 1-2 inches deep with the buds pointing upward.
- **Water and Sun:** Ginger prefers partial to full shade. Keep the soil consistently moist but avoid waterlogging. Ginger plants will die under direct heat from the sun.
- **Harvesting:** Ginger takes about 8-10 months to mature. You can start harvesting small pieces as needed after a few months, but for the full rhizome, wait until the plant starts dying back.

Ginger is not only a flavorful addition to many dishes but also a powerful herb with numerous medicinal properties. As always, use in moderation and consult a healthcare professional for therapeutic uses.

Goldenseal

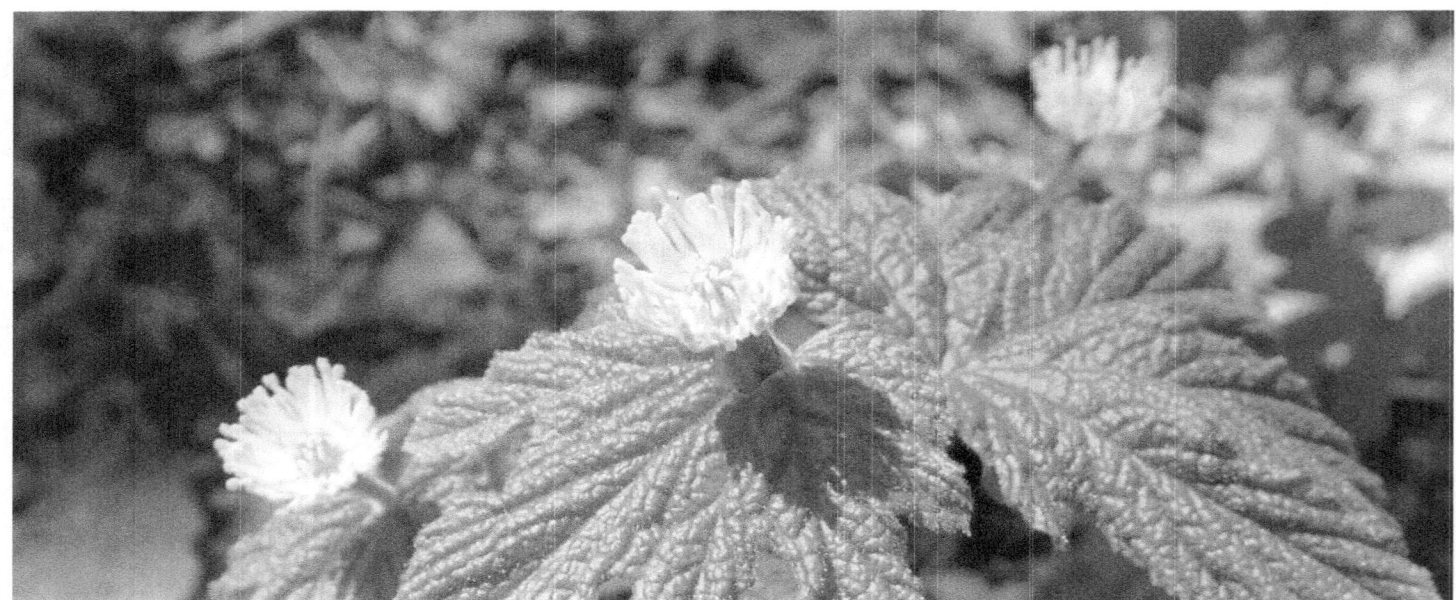

Goldenseal is a plant with flower, it is commonly found in North America. Goldenseal has a yellowish root underground and above the ground the stem is hairy and purple in color. The plant helps fight a lot of health issues including ulcers.

Botanical Name: Hydrastis canadensis

Family: Ranunculaceae

Common Names: Golden-seal, Yellow Root, Orangeroot, Ground Raspberry

Medicinal Properties:

Goldenseal is a woodland herb native to North America and has a long history of use among Native American tribes due to its therapeutic attributes. The herb has multiple benefits for the human body. It helps develop a stronger immunity.

- **Anti-microbial:** The alkaloid berberine in goldenseal has shown effectiveness against various bacteria, fungi, and protozoa. It protects the organs from different bacteria, it also prevents fungus from spreading within the body while curing the fungus from its root.
- **Digestive Aid:** Traditionally used to help with stomach ailments, from ulcers to diarrhea. Like multiple herbs, goldenseal helps with gut health and stomach issues.
- **Mucous Membrane Soother:** Goldenseal is often used to soothe inflamed mucus membranes of the nose, throat, and digestive tract. It helps people with sinus as it eases the process of breathing by clearing or thinning the mucus wall on the pipes.
- **Immune System Boost:** It is believed to have properties that help boost the immune system. Improved gut health means improved immunity, goldenseal has properties and chemicals that help strengthen the immunity.
- **Liver Function:** Goldenseal helps in detoxifying the liver, making it fat free and performing its functions efficiently.

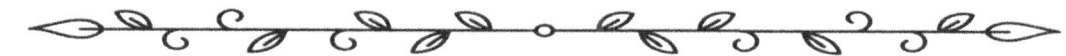

Uses as a Herbal Antibiotic:

- **Respiratory Infections:** Often combined with echinacea to treat colds and influenza, goldenseal is known to help ease the breathing process and relax inflammations.
- **Skin Infections:** Used topically, goldenseal can be effective for fungal infections and other skin irritations. Though, it is advised to use it with a mix of other relaxing and cooling herbs for better efficiency.
- **Digestive Infections:** Taken orally, goldenseal can help in addressing bacterial infections in the digestive system. It clears the GI tract of all the harmful bacteria and lets it pass out of the body without inflicting harm to the digestive health.

Precautions:

- **Pregnancy and Lactation:** It is an herb that can cause harm to the pregnant body and even the foetus. It is also not advised to take goldenseal if you are a feeding mother.
- **Blood Pressure:** It might interfere with blood pressure control; those with hypertension should be cautious. Golden-seal has properties that can increase the blood pressure, so if you are a blood pressure patient, it is advised to take golden-seal under strict supervision and on recommendation of a physician.
- **Blood Sugar Levels:** It might lower blood sugar levels, which could interfere with diabetes management. Goldenseal is known to negatively affect the blood sugar level, so do not take it on an empty stomach or right after the blood sugar medicine.

Side Effects:

- Nausea or vomiting
- Irritation when applied to the skin
- Digestive distress
- Nervous system issues when consumed in large quantities

How to Grow Goldenseal:

Goldenseal is a woodland plant that thrives in shaded, moist environments. It needs to be sheltered from direct sunlight.

- **Starting:** Golden-seal seeds require stratification. Before planting, store them in a moist medium in a refrigerator for several months.
- **Soil and Sun:** Goldenseal prefers rich, well-draining soil with a slightly acidic to neutral pH. It requires partial to full shade. A higher pH sol can hinder its growth.
- **Planting:** Seeds or rhizome cuttings can be planted in the spring, spaced 6-8 inches apart.
- **Watering:** Regular watering is essential but ensure the soil doesn't become waterlogged.
- **Harvesting:** The roots are the primary medicinal part and can be harvested in the fall of the third or fourth year.

Growing goldenseal requires patience, as it takes a few years to mature. Given its declining populations in the wild due to over-harvesting, cultivating goldenseal can help conserve this valuable plant. As always, consult a healthcare professional before using goldenseal for medicinal purposes.

Oregano

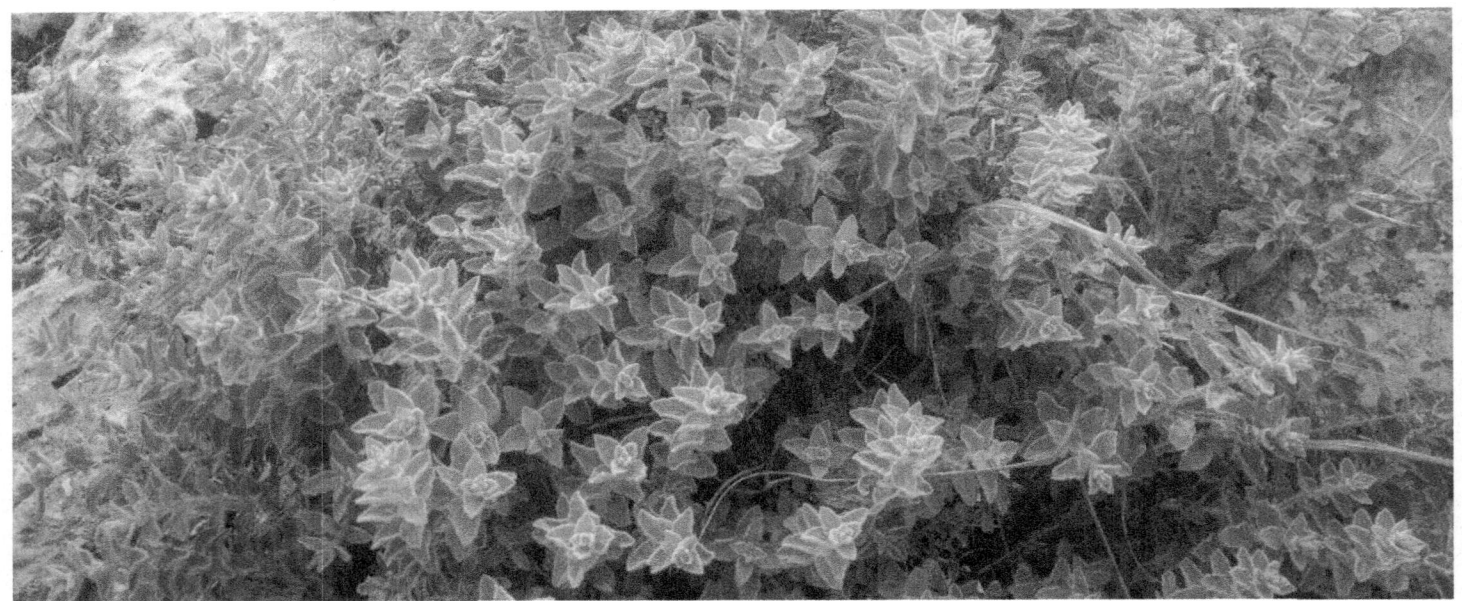

Oregano is also an herb used for curing illnesses alongside being used in different recipes. It also can be used as an oil for a more infused and potent elixir to treat an ailment. The plant of oregano is common and can be grown at home under normal climate and with little care and look-after.

Botanical Name: Origanum vulgare

Family: Lamiaceae

Common Names: Oregano, Wild Marjoram, Sweet Marjoram

Medicinal Properties:

Oregano isn't just a popular culinary herb; it has long been revered for its potential health benefits. It has been used over centuries to treat problems related to inflammation, gut health, releasing toxins from the body, etc.

- **Anti-microbial:** Oregano oil, particularly its component Carvacrol, has been demonstrated to have strong antibacterial and anti-fungal properties. A person with infections and recurring diseases can use oregano oil to kill the harmful bacteria and stop the fungus from spreading at a faster pace.
- **Antioxidant:** The herb is rich in antioxidants, which help combat free radicals in the body. toxins and dangerous chemicals are treated by oregano to not impact the body in a negative manner.
- **Anti-inflammatory:** Components like terpenes, rosmarinic acid, and thymol within oregano act as inflammation-reducing agents. It helps with keeping the organs relaxed and aid the organs in performing its functions seamlessly.
- **Digestive Aid:** Traditional uses include settling digestive disorders and stimulating the appetite. For someone who isn't on a normal weight scale and has to gain weight, the most effective way is to do it through consumption of healthy food. consumption of oregano increases the appetite to help you eat more.

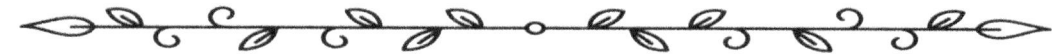

Uses as an Herbal Antibiotic:

- **Respiratory Infections:** Oregano oil is often recommended as a natural remedy for bacterial and viral respiratory infections.
- **Skin Infections:** Applied topically, diluted oregano oil can combat certain fungal infections and skin irritations. It can also release any inflammation of the joints.
- **Digestive Ailments:** It's believed to help ward off harmful gut bacteria and parasites. It kills off the stomach worms that are dangerous for the health and can ruin the gastrointestinal health.

Precautions:

- **Pregnancy:** High doses or concentrated supplements should be avoided during pregnancy. This is a general rule, oregano is, though, a safe herb but overuse can negatively affect the pregnancy.
- **Blood Thinners:** Oregano might increase the risk of bleeding in individuals on anticoagulant medications. Most herbs have the tendency to thin the blood out, so it is not advised to take any hard or concentrated herb while a person is already on blood thinning medication.
- **Allergies:** People sensitive to plants in the Lamiaceae family (like basil, lavender, mint) might also be allergic to oregano.

Side Effects:

- Stomach upset when consumed in large amounts.
- Skin irritation when applied topically without dilution.
- Possible lowering of blood sugar levels.

How to Grow Oregano:

Oregano is a perennial herb and growing it can provide a fresh supply year after year.

- **Planting:** You can start oregano from seeds, cuttings, or purchased plants. Plant them about 8 to 10 inches apart in your garden.
- **Soil and Sun:** Oregano prefers well-draining soil and full sun. However, it can also tolerate light shade.
- **Watering:** Water regularly, but make sure not to over-water. Oregano is drought-resistant once established.
- **Pruning:** Pinch or trim the tops of the plant during the growing season to encourage a bushier and more compact plant.
- **Harvesting:** Pick oregano leaves as needed. For the most robust flavor, harvest just before the plant blooms, which is typically in early summer.

With its fragrant leaves and robust flavor, oregano is a delight to grow and beneficial for health. As with all herbs, it's vital to use it thoughtfully and consult with a healthcare professional if considering its medicinal uses.

Thyme

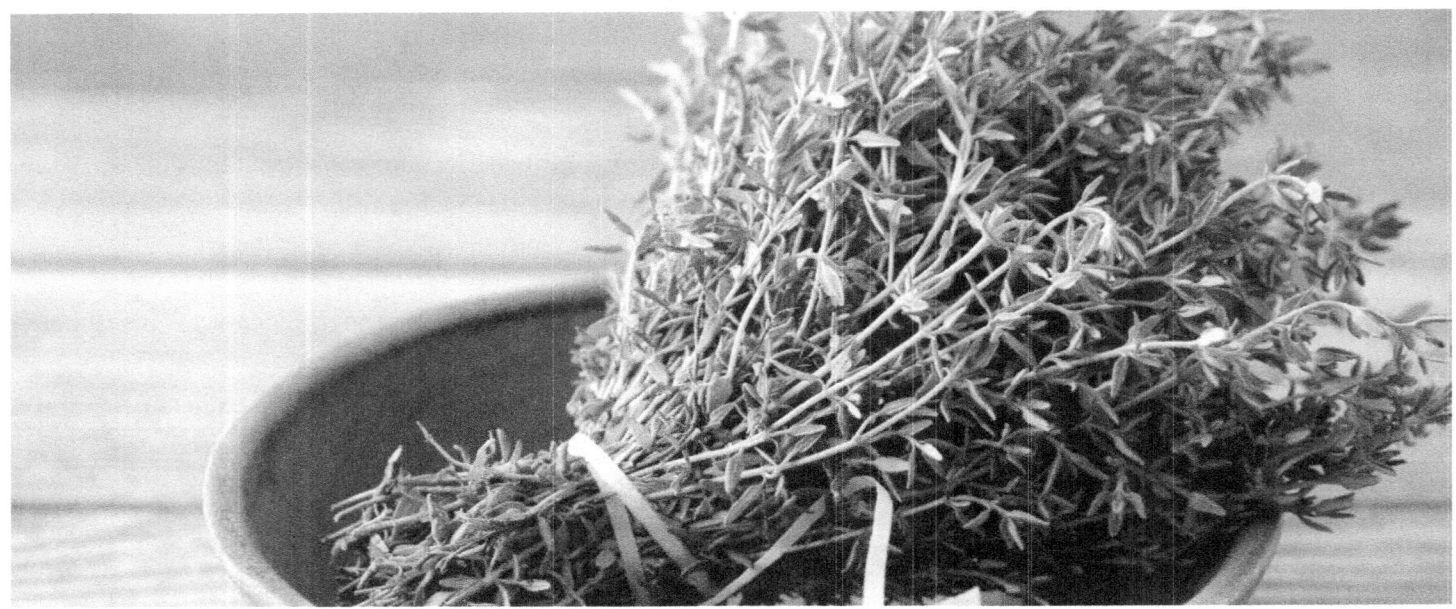

Thyme is a cherished and well-known herb. It has been found in the books of early healers and cooking experts to be used in healing and cooking alike. Thyme gives a lot of flavor and aroma to the food; it also aids with ailing people's treatments.

Botanical Name: Thymus vulgaris

Family: Lamiaceae

Common Names: Common Thyme, Garden Thyme

Medicinal Properties:

Thyme is not just a culinary staple; it's also been used medicinally for thousands of years to treat multiple issues related to human health.

- **Anti-microbial:** Thymol, a primary chemical compound in thyme, has powerful antiseptic and antibacterial properties. It prevents bacteria from spreading in the body. It is a powerful agent that kills the bacteria from the root and stops it from resurfacing.
- **Expectorant:** Thyme can help loosen mucus in the respiratory tract, making it beneficial for coughs and congestion. It helps make it clear and makes the windpipes easier to breathe.
- **Antioxidant:** The herb boasts high levels of antioxidants, which help combat free radicals in the body. toxins and other harmful chemicals that float free in our body are dismissed by thyme and excreted through the proper channel.
- **Anti-inflammatory:** Thyme has been used to alleviate inflammation, particularly for conditions like sore throats. Thyme helps reduce bacterial inflammation and the mucus wall to a great extent.

Uses as an Herbal Antibiotic:

- **Respiratory Issues:** Thyme tea or syrup is traditionally used to relieve coughs, bronchitis, and other respiratory problems. Syrups with thyme and other herbal medicines are easily available if one doesn't want to make syrup or tea.

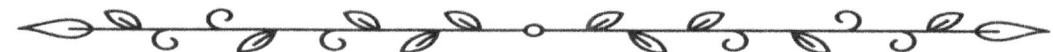

- **Oral Health:** Due to its antibacterial properties, thyme is sometimes found in natural mouthwashes to combat bad breath and oral pathogens. Thyme improves gum health and prevents cavities from building on teeth.
- **Skin Infections:** Thyme oil, when diluted, can be applied topically to treat minor cuts, scrapes, and acne due to its antiseptic properties. It has benefits to treat skin issues that lie under the epidermis.

Precautions:
- **Pregnancy and Breastfeeding:** It's best to limit medicinal amounts of thyme during pregnancy and while breastfeeding.
- **Blood Pressure:** High doses might lower blood pressure, so people with low blood pressure or those taking medications should be cautious. It is best to consult a physician or your medical practitioner before using thyme as a medication.
- **Thyroid:** High amounts of thyme might affect thyroid hormone levels.

Side Effects:
- Some people might experience gastrointestinal discomfort when consumed in large amounts.
- Possible allergic reactions, mainly when applied topically.
- Over-consumption might lead to headaches or dizziness.

How to Grow Thyme:
Thyme is a versatile and hardy perennial herb that grows relatively quickly.
- **Planting:** You can start thyme from seeds, cuttings, or nursery transplants. Plant them about 12 to 24 inches apart. It is not necessary to plant thyme from seeds. You can plant it from a small thyme plant or a bunch of thyme.
- **Soil and Sun:** Thyme prefers well-draining soil and full sun but can tolerate light shade. It is, though, necessary to give it direct sunlight every few days, if not daily.
- **Watering:** Water regularly until the plant is established. After that, thyme is drought-tolerant and needs less frequent watering.
- **Pruning:** Regular pruning, especially after flowering, helps to keep the plant bushy and healthy. It is best to prune keeping in mind the general rules of pruning. Do not pluck most of the leaves from a single branch to keep it healthy and growing at its maximum capacity.
- **Harvesting:** Thyme can be harvested anytime, but for the best flavor, consider harvesting just before it flowers.

Incorporating thyme into your garden adds culinary versatility and medicinal benefits. As with any herb used for therapeutic purposes, ensure you use thyme judiciously and consult a healthcare professional when considering more potent or frequent usage.

Turmeric

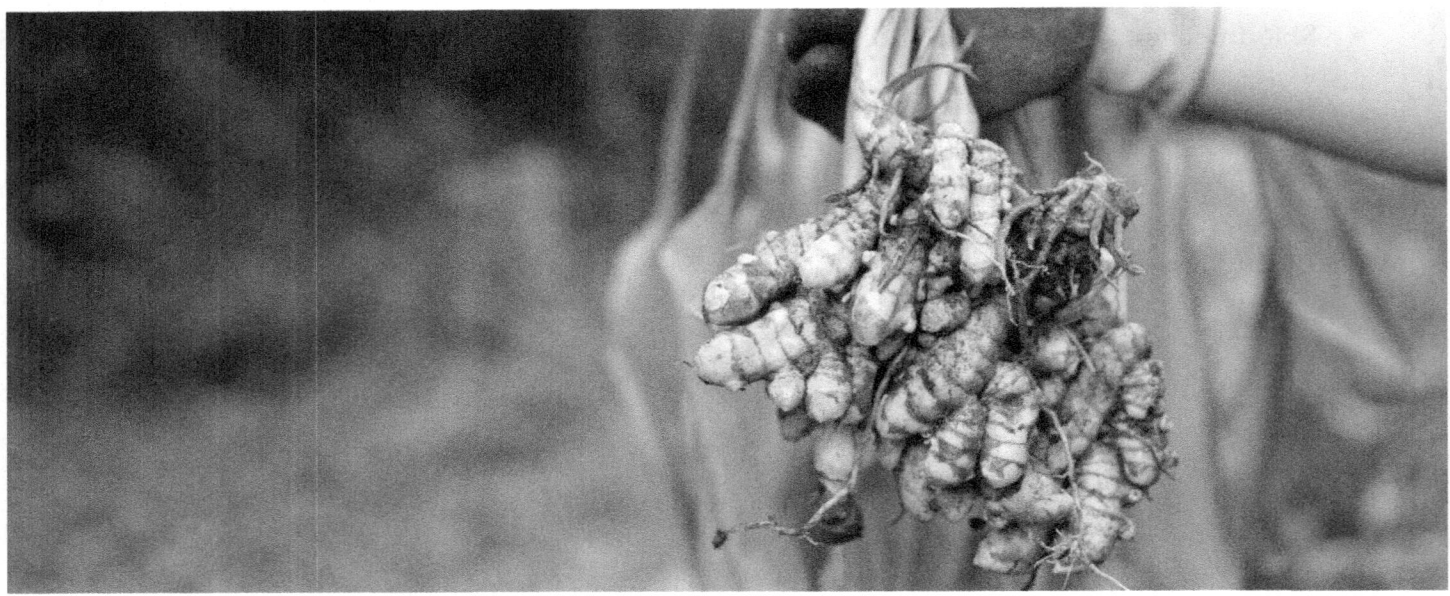

Turmeric is one of the most common herbs used for medicinal purposes worldwide. It is known for its multiple health benefits, from curing cuts and scrapes to relieving joint aches. Turmeric originated from Asia but can now be found in most of the countries. It, however, does not flourish in extremely cold climates.

Botanical Name: Curcuma longa

Family: Zingiberaceae

Common Names: Turmeric, Indian Saffron, Haldi

Medicinal Properties:

Turmeric, a staple in many Asian cuisines, has been utilized medicinally for over 4,000 years:

- **Anti-inflammatory:** Curcumin, the active component in turmeric, has potent anti-inflammatory effects which can rival some anti-inflammatory drugs. It provides a soothing effect to areas that are inflamed.
- **Antioxidant:** Turmeric not only contains antioxidants but also boosts the body's antioxidant enzymes. It gives the body a cellular makeover, releasing the intoxicated cells and producing new cells.
- **Brain Functionality:** Curcumin has been shown to increase brain levels of brain-derived neurotrophic factor, a type of growth hormone that functions in the brains. Turmeric promotes a healthy brain functionality. It opens up the cortex's and keeps the mind in a peaceful place taking it out from an over-exerted flight or fight situation or overthinking.
- **Antiviral and Antibacterial:** Turmeric displays antiviral and antibacterial properties, which can help fight infections. Turmeric can be administered in multiple ways to help kill the bacteria or the virus that is present in the body.

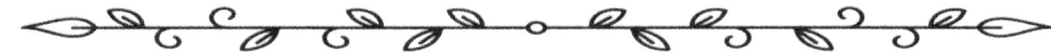

Uses as an Herbal Antibiotic:

Wound Healing: Turmeric paste can be applied to cuts and wounds to prevent bacterial infections. Turmeric can also be drunk in milk or in plain water as tea to cure many issues like aches, cold, flu, sneezing, cough, etc.

- **Digestive Health:** It promotes digestion and reduce symptoms of bloating and gas. Turmeric used in food also helps with keeping stomach bacteria and worms in check.
- **Respiratory Infections:** Turmeric milk or "Golden Milk" is a traditional remedy for coughs and colds in many cultures. The turmeric milk is given even if a person has some minor injuries, it is said to cure the internal injuries that cannot be seen on the surface.
- **Joint and Muscle Pain:** Its anti-inflammatory properties make it a natural remedy for arthritic pain and muscle inflammation. Turmeric is one of the best remedies present for inflammation. It treats inflammation from the root to make sure it is gone for a long time.

Precautions:

- **Gallbladder Issues:** Those with gallstones or bile duct obstructions should avoid turmeric as it may exacerbate the issue. turmeric takes a while to digest as it mostly gets absorbed in the blood stream. It is better to avoid it if you have stones in the gallbladder or other gestational issues.
- **Diabetes:** Turmeric might lower blood sugar, so those with diabetes or on diabetes medication should monitor their levels closely.

Side Effects:

- High doses or prolonged use can cause gastrointestinal problems like GERD or stomach ulcers.
- This is very rare, but still can happen, allergic reactions, like rashes or hives. One must do a small taste test before incorporating turmeric in their diet of medication.
- May cause nausea, diarrhea, or dizziness in some individuals.

How to Grow Turmeric:

Turmeric is grown from rhizomes and prefers warm, humid conditions.

- **Planting:** Start with a turmeric rhizome from a nursery or organic grocery store. Break it into smaller pieces, ensuring each has a bud or two.
- **Soil and Sun:** Turmeric prefers well-draining, slightly acidic soil. It thrives in partial sun or light shade.
- **Watering:** Water moderately. The soil should be kept moist but not waterlogged.
- **Harvesting:** Turmeric typically takes 8-10 months to mature. The leaves and stems will start to turn brown and dry. At this point, you can dig up the rhizomes.
- **Curing:** After harvesting, boil the rhizomes, then dry them for several days. Once dried, they can be ground into turmeric powder.

Turmeric is not only a culinary treasure but also a potent herbal remedy. It's crucial to use it wisely and always consult with a healthcare professional for therapeutic purposes, especially if taken in supplement form or for extended periods.

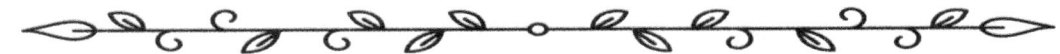

Summary

There are multiple herbs that have been discussed in detail along with its uses and how to avoid any negative effects it may have on a person health.

- Echinacea is also known as Coneflower; it is mostly found in Eastern and Central North America. It has multiple health benefits, like, it strengthens immunity, treats bronchitis, is good for sinusitis, etc. There are a few side effects that must be kept in mind, like, it thins the blood so it should not be taken with blood thinners.

- Garlic is a natural remedy for many illnesses and has been used for medicinal purposes for more than centuries now. It benefits sore throat and helps clear mucus. It has blood thinning properties and should not be overused by people with cardiovascular issues. It is great for kids with sinus issues and breathing problems. It can cause skin irritation if applied topically.

- Ginger has an acidic and spicy flavor to it. It is an ingredient in many recipes, but its medicinal benefits are amazing. It calms the mind and relaxes the body. Other than that, it has multiple benefits for women from reducing period cramps to treating PCOs.

- Goldenseal may take a lot of time and care to grow but the results and healing properties are worth it. It helps in curing ulcers and helps with digestive health. Although, it is not advised to be used above a certain limit for pregnant women or feeding mothers.

- Oregano oil is used to treat fungus and inflammation. It also stimulates appetite to help gain body mass and build muscle. Oregano is known as a great herb to add to your food, it also has multiple benefits for the body internally.

- Thyme is an incredible herb that can elevate the flavor and aroma of your food. Thyme also has antimicrobial properties, and it helps loosen the mucus wall from the throat and windpipe. It has a higher level of antioxidants, making the body lose toxins easily.

- Turmeric is the easiest yet the most beneficial herb we can have. It can heal internal injuries, it can soothe skin issues by applying it topically, the benefits and uses are endless. It is advised not to use blood thinners.

Practical Applications:
Herbal Antibiotics for Common Ailments

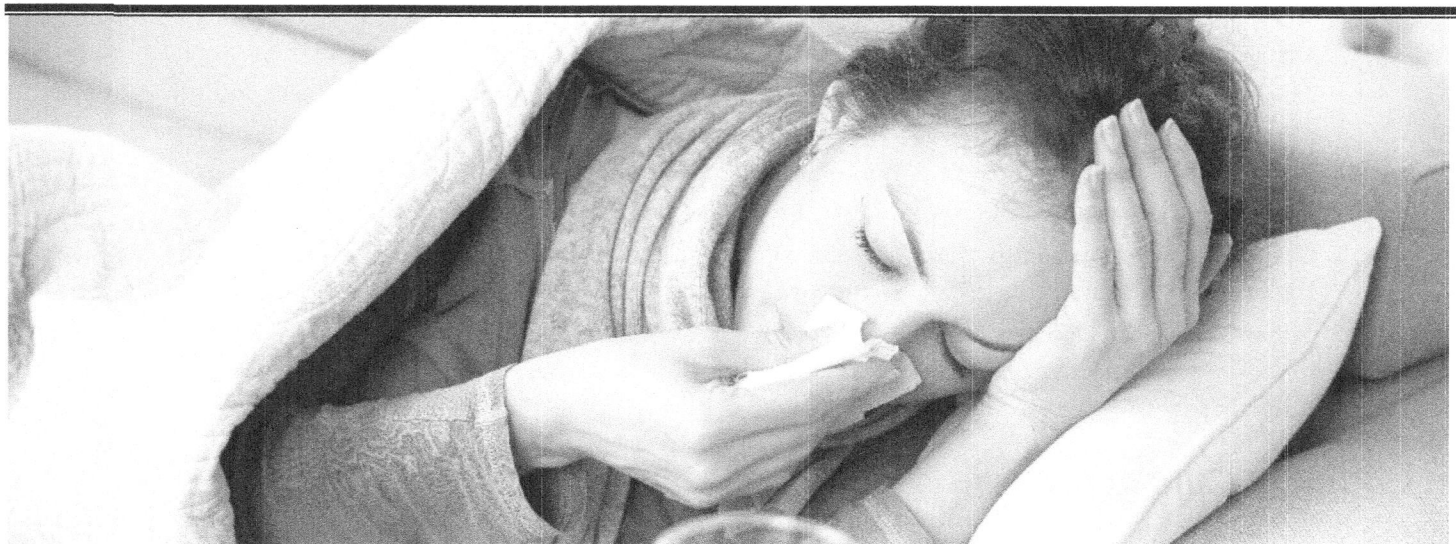

Using herbal antibiotics to treat common illnesses is a natural and efficient way to stimulate your immune system and promote recovery. Before beginning any treatment, getting advice from a medical expert familiar with herbal remedies is necessary.

Do your research and pick the appropriate herbs, such as garlic, echinacea, golden-seal, or oregano oil, known to have antibiotic characteristics. The potency of each herb may vary, and it may be available in various formats, such as teas, tinctures, capsules, or infused oils. Ensure you know each herb's recommended dosage and any possible negative effects.

When taking herbal medicines, consistency is essential. Utilize the herbal antibiotics following the advised dosage and schedule. Maintain the course of treatment and give the herbs adequate time to take effect.

To boost your immune system when using herbal antibiotics, maintain a healthy lifestyle. Eat a balanced diet, regularly exercise, get enough sleep, and drink lots of water.

Keep a watchful eye on your symptoms while taking herbal antibiotics. Consult a medical expert if your issue doesn't get better or worsens. They can provide you with further direction and modify your treatment as needed.

Herbal antibiotics may help treat common illnesses but shouldn't replace prescription medical care for serious or persistent disorders. Seek expert guidance to ensure safe and suitable use. In the end, the prudent and knowledgeable use of herbal antibiotics can offer a natural means of treating common illnesses while promoting your general health.

Introduction to Practical Applications

Practical applications are crucial to use herbal antibiotics to treat common illnesses effectively. Practical applications enable people to make informed judgments about their health by giving comprehensive information on each typical ailment and its related herbal antibiotics. It enables individuals to successfully use herbal antibiotics to support their well-being while exploring natural alternatives with assurance.

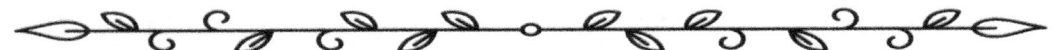

You can determine each herbal antibiotic's useful uses in treating different medical conditions by learning the particular traits and capabilities of each one.

Detailed instructions on utilizing herbal antibiotics to treat a particular common sickness are included in each condition description. The following details will be provided:

- The common sickness, its symptoms, and potential causes will be described at the beginning of the profile.
- The herbal antibiotics proven successful in treating that ailment are then included as recommended herbs. For example, herbs like thyme or eucalyptus may be suggested if the condition is a respiratory illness.
- The profile will describe the many herbal antibiotics available and how to prepare them. This can include directions for creating an herbal tincture, brewing a tea, or utilizing an infused oil.
- Detailed instructions on the right amount to take and how often to take a natural antibiotic will be given. This guarantees the right herb dosage to increase potency while preventing negative effects.
- The profile might also recommend supplementary treatments or lifestyle modifications that can aid the healing process even more. These could include nutritional advice, stress-reduction tactics, or other herbal supplements to take in addition to antibiotics.

Common Cold and Flu

Various herbs might offer comfort and help your immune system when using herbal antibiotics to treat the common cold and flu. Herbal antibiotics holds a significant value when it comes to treating common cold and flu and shows effective results in a short period of time,

Here is a list of herbs to use, instructions for preparing them, and dosage suggestions:

Echinacea: Echinacea is a well-liked herb known for enhancing the immune system. It may decrease the intensity and length of colds and flu. Echinacea comes in various forms, including tablets, capsules, teas, and tinctures. For precise instructions, refer to a healthcare practitioner or the dosage recommendations on the product's packaging.

Ginger: Ginger naturally fights bacteria and viruses, which can assist with cold and flu symptoms. Take a piece of ginger-which should be fresh, grate it, and steep it for 10 to 15 minutes in hot water to make ginger tea. For additional calming effects, incorporate honey and lemon. Take this tea several times daily to ease sore throats and clear up congestion.

Elderberry: The powerful antiviral effects of elderberry are widely known. To strengthen your immune system and lower your chance of contracting an illness during the cold and flu season, elderberry syrup or capsules are commonly accessible. The product's dose recommendations should be followed, or you can seek medical advice.

Garlic: Garlic's potent antibacterial capabilities can assist in battling the flu and cold viruses. You can eat raw garlic by including it in your diet—for example, by blending it into sauces, salad dressings, or soups. Alternatively, garlic supplements can be consumed as instructed on the label or by a healthcare provider's prescription.

Thyme: Thyme can help reduce congestion brought on by a cold or the flu and is a great expectorant. Steep dried thyme leaves in boiling water for 10 to 15 minutes to make thyme tea. Tea should be strained and consumed warmly. Lemon and honey can be added for added advantages. Drink this tea two to three times daily to relieve congestion and coughing.

It's vital to remember that herbal antibiotics should be used cautiously, just like any other medication. To ensure the herbs are secure and suitable, consult a doctor, especially if you have any other health issues or are taking other medications.

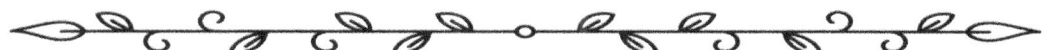

Additionally, keep in mind to drink enough water while sick. Drink plenty of liquids, such as homemade soup, hot water with honey and lemon, or herbal teas (such as chamomile or peppermint). This promotes the healing process and keeps your body hydrated.

Taking herbal antibiotics to treat the common cold and flu can help your immune system and relieve you. You can consume herbs like echinacea, ginger, elderberry, garlic, and thyme as teas, pills, or as part of your diet. To ensure safe and efficient use, adhere to recommended dosages and consult a healthcare practitioner. To encourage a quick recovery, drink plenty of water, take the medicines on time, get plenty of rest, and eat healthfully.

Urinary Tract Infections

A natural and alternative method of treating this widespread problem is to use herbal antibiotics to treat urinary tract infections (UTIs). Herbal medications with antibacterial qualities and possible benefits for treating UTIs include bearberry, goldenseal, marshmallow root, and dandelion root. To get a precise diagnosis and advice, speaking with a medical expert is essential. This overview of herbal antibiotics for treating UTIs includes information on selecting suitable herbs, preparation techniques, and suggested dosages. It is significant to remember that these treatments should only be used when necessary and should not replace medical care.

However, speaking with a medical expert before utilizing herbal therapies is crucial, particularly if you have a UTI. Following are some herbal antibiotics useful for treating urinary tract infections:

Bearberry (Uva Ursi): Bearberry (Uva Ursi) is a popular plant for UTIs due to its antibacterial qualities. It contains an element called arbutin, which, when transformed into hydroquinone in the urinary system, aids in suppressing bacterial growth. Bearberry should not be taken for an extended period, and dosage recommendations should be strictly heeded.

Golden-seal: Used to treat UTIs, golden-seal is renowned for its antibacterial and anti-inflammatory effects. The active ingredient in goldenseal, berberine, is thought to have antibacterial properties.

Marshmallow root: Known for its calming effects, it may help relieve UTI symptoms, including frequent urination or burning. As a supplement rather than an actual antibiotic, it is frequently utilized. For advice on the dose, seek the advice of a medical practitioner.

Dandelion root: The diuretic qualities of the dandelion root can aid in clearing bacteria from the urinary tract. It is also regarded as an immune system enhancer that helps the body fight off illnesses. Consuming dandelion root for treat urinary tract infections is one of the best herbal antibiotics.

It is essential to choose the right herbal antibiotic for the required treatment. For advice on choosing the right herbs, properly preparing them, and adhering to suggested dosages, speak with a healthcare expert. When necessary, these remedies should not be used in place of medical care; they also need to be under professional supervision.

Dosage Recommendations:

Following established dosage guidelines and properly preparing all of these herbs before using them is crucial. These guidelines can change based on the herb and a person's needs. Here is a general rule of thumb:

- Always abide by the directions with the particular herbal product, as they may differ.
- It is important to adhere to the suggested dosage because going overboard could have negative consequences. Also take the dosage timely.

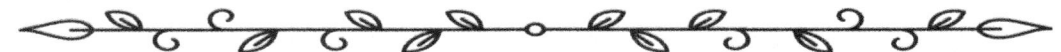

- Typically, herbal antibiotics come in tinctures, pills, or teas. For information on recommended dosage, refer to the product label.
- Consult a licensed herbalist to determine the right brewing time and dosage if you use herbal tea.

Remember that not everyone will get the same results or experience success with herbal therapies, and severe UTIs may necessitate medical attention. For accurate diagnosis and advice on the best course of action for your particular circumstance, it is imperative that you speak with a healthcare expert.

Skin Infections

Using herbal antibiotics to treat skin infections entails employing natural plant-based therapies to combat infection and encourage recovery. It's crucial to seek advice from a skilled herbalist or healthcare provider before using herbal antibiotics to treat skin infections to confirm that the treatment is appropriate for your condition or circumstance. Even though people have used herbal treatments for ages, it's important to be cautious and refrain from self-diagnosis and self-medication.

However, the following are some generally applicable herbs and suggestions:

The calendula plant (Calendula officinalis)

- Its antibacterial and anti-inflammatory qualities are well known.
- Calendula oil preparation involves steeping dried calendula flowers in any oil, such as olive oil or coconut oil, for a few weeks before straining.
- 2-3 times a day, topically apply the oil to the troubled regions.

Melaleuca alternifolia, or tea tree

- Possesses potent anti-fungal and antibacterial activities.
- Apply tea tree essential oil to the affected area many times each day by dilution in a carrier oil like coconut oil.
- Not to be consumed is tea tree oil.

Allium sativum, or garlic

- Garlic has strong antibacterial abilities.
- Crush some fresh garlic cloves, then make a paste and apply it directly to the infection. Before cleaning, wrap it in a fresh bandage and let it sit for a few hours.
- Creams or ointments made with garlic extract can be used as an alternative.

(Echinacea purpurea) Echinacea

- It supports immunological health and has antibacterial properties.
- Topically apply echinacea cream or ointment several times daily to the afflicted area.

Manuka Honey

- Manuka honey demonstrates strong antibacterial properties.
- After applying a thin layer of medical grade manuka honey, a clean bandage should be placed over the region. 2-3 times every day, change the bandage and reapply honey.
- Consult a professional for help since usage guidelines can vary.

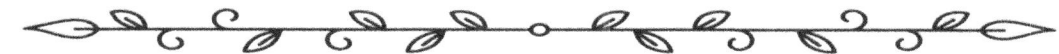

Aloe Vera

- It is well known for its ability to reduce swelling and heal wounds.
- Apply the aloe Vera leaf gel straight to the treatment area. Before rinsing, leave it on for a few hours.
- Repeat a minimum of three times daily until the infection clears up.

(Azadirachta indica) Neem:

- Neem possesses anti-inflammatory, anti-fungal, and anti-microbial activities.
- Neem oil can be directly applied or diluted with carrier oil and applied to the afflicted region.
- 1-2 times per day.

(Curcuma longa) Turmeric

- Turmeric possesses antibacterial and anti-inflammatory properties.
- To make a paste, combine turmeric powder with either water or coconut oil.
- After applying the paste and leaving it on for 15 to 20 minutes, rinse the area with water.
- Take it three or more times daily.

Mahonia aquifolium, often known as Oregon Grape Root.

- It possesses anti-inflammatory and anti-microbial activities.
- Creating herbal oil for many weeks, infuse dried Oregon grape root in a carrier oil like coconut or olive oil. After straining, store it in a dark glass bottle.
- 2-3 times each day, apply the oil directly to the diseased region and gently massage it in.

Depending on the nature and severity of the infection, different dosage recommendations and preparations may be needed. Always seek personalized guidance from a medical expert or herbalist to ensure safe use. Seek quick medical assistance if the infection gets worse or continues.

Respiratory Infections

Incorporating herbal medications to treat respiratory infections entails using homeopathic treatments to boost the body's immune system and ward against infections. Speaking with a medical expert or a licensed herbalist for particular advice depending on your circumstances while utilizing herbal antibiotics to treat respiratory infections is essential. Here are some often-used herbs and some basic suggestions:

(Echinacea purpurea) Echinacea

- Echinacea is renowned for its antibacterial and immune-stimulating qualities.
- It is available in various forms, including teas, tinctures, and capsules.
- Follow the suggested dosage listed on the product label or the advice of a health care provider.

(Salvia officinalis) Sage:

- It has antiviral and antibacterial activities.
- Sage tea steers 1-2 tablespoons of dried sage leaves for 10-15 minutes in a cup of boiling water. Drink it several times daily after straining.
- Follow the directions on any sage products, such as lozenges or throat sprays.

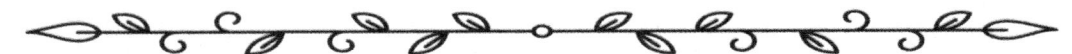

(Thymus vulgaris) Thyme

- Thyme contains substances with antibacterial properties.
- Two teaspoons of dried thyme leaves should be boiled for 8-10 minutes in a cup of boiling water. 2-3 times a day, strain it and consume.
- Thyme essential oil can be applied directly or diluted and inhaled through steam. However, for the proper dilution ratios and techniques, seek professional advice.
- Has antibacterial and decongestant qualities.

(Mentha x piperita) Peppermint

- One to two tablespoons of dried peppermint leaves steeped in boiling water for ten minutes will yield peppermint tea. 2-3 times a day, strain it and consume.
- You can diffuse peppermint essential oil or apply it topically after diluting it. Consult a specialist for safe usage advice.

(Allium sativum) Garlic

- It has antibacterial and immune-boosting qualities.
- Eat much fresh garlic or follow the directions on any supplements you take.
- Crush a clove of raw garlic and combine it with honey or olive oil. Take this mixture two or three times daily.

(Origanum vulgare) Oregano:

- It consists of substances with potent antibacterial activity.
- Use oregano oil directly on the chest or throat area by taking oregano oil capsules or combining it with a carrier oil and a few drops of essential oil.
- Utilize the product's instructions or consult a specialist.

Glycyrrhiza glabra, also known as licorice root

- It has antibacterial and anti-inflammatory properties.
- Soak 1-2 tablespoons of dried licorice root for 10-15 minutes in boiling water to make licorice root tea. 2-3 times a day, strain it and consume.
- It is also possible to utilize throat lozenges or licorice root supplements. Observe the suggested dosage that is given.

Always check to ensure you have no allergies to these herbs and be wary of any potential drug interactions or health issues.

Remember that different respiratory illnesses have different degrees of severity, and some can call for medical attention. Although they shouldn't be taken in place of proper medical care, herbal antibiotics can be used as additional assistance. A treatment plan, which is personalized based on your unique condition, can be obtained by consulting a medical practitioner.

Remember to practice excellent hygiene, get enough rest, and stay hydrated when battling respiratory infections. If symptoms get worse, you should see a doctor.

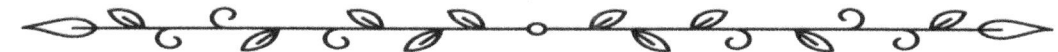

Digestive Issues

In a holistic approach to treating digestion problems, herbal antibiotics may offer comfort and maintain digestive health. For specific advice on your condition while utilizing herbal antibiotics to treat digestive disorders, speak with a healthcare provider or a licensed herbalist. Here are some often-used herbs and some basic suggestions:

Mentha x piperita, peppermint:

- It relieves indigestion, gas, and other digestive issues.
- One to two tablespoons of dried peppermint leaves steeped in boiling water for ten minutes will yield peppermint tea. 2-3 times a day, strain it and consume.
- You can also take peppermint oil or capsules, but for the right dosage, talk to a doctor.

Zingiber officinale, or ginger

- It improves digestion and eases indigestion and motion sickness.
- Around two teaspoons of freshly grated ginger should be cooked in boiling water for ten minutes to make ginger tea. 2-3 times a day, strain it and consume.
- You can also use ginger supplements or candies but utilize the correct dosage.

Matricaria chamomilla, or chamomile:

- It aids in reducing bloating and indigestion while soothing the digestive tract.
- To make chamomile tea, two to three tablespoons of dried chamomile flowers should be steeped in boiling water for ten minutes. 2-3 times a day, strain it and consume.
- You can also use chamomile pills or tinctures. Consult a professional for advice on the right dosage.

Foeniculum vulgare, or fennel:

- It reduces bloating, gas, and discomfort in the digestive system.
- 1-2 tablespoons of crushed fennel seeds steeped in boiling water for 10 minutes will yield fennel tea. 2-3 times a day, strain it and consume.
- There may be fennel supplements or capsules on the market. Observe the suggested dosage that is given.

Ulmus rubra, the slippery elm

- It soothes the digestive tract and aids in reducing inflammation and heartburn.
- Combine 1-2 teaspoons of slippery elm powder with water to make a paste. Eat it after meals.
- You can also use slippery elm lozenges or pills as indicated.

Althaea officinalis, sometimes known as marshmallow root

- It forms a shield over the digestive tract, easing gastrointestinal discomfort and symptoms like acid re-flux.
- Soak 1-2 tablespoons of dried marshmallow root for 10-15 minutes in boiling water to make marshmallow root tea. 2-3 times a day, strain it and consume.
- There may also be supplements or tinctures made from marshmallow root. Observe the suggested dosage that is given.

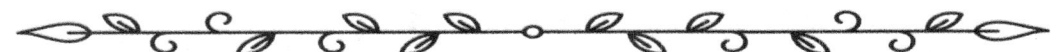

Keeping this in mind, it's crucial to identify the underlying source of your digestive problems so you can treat them effectively. Always speak with a doctor or herbalist for specific guidance, especially if you're taking medication or have a chronic disease.

Different dosage suggestions and formulations may be appropriate depending on a person's situation and the seriousness of the digestive problem. It's best to consult a specialist for sound advice.

In addition to herbal medicines, good digestive health can be achieved and promoted by eating a balanced diet, eating more frequently, drinking enough water, and controlling stress. Seek quick medical attention for an accurate diagnosis if symptoms intensify or continue to persist.

Preventive Measures and Boosting Immunity

Herbal antibiotics can be useful tools for preventing illness and naturally boosting immunity. Herbal medicines offer a wider spectrum of immune-boosting and antibacterial qualities than synthetic antibiotics, which treat specific illnesses. They can improve general well-being, assist the body's defense mechanisms, and lower the risk of several infections.

Many plants have traditionally been utilized for their antibacterial, antiviral, and immune-stimulating characteristics. Several herbs, including echinacea, garlic, ginger, turmeric, and Andrographis, have come to be known for their potential immune-stimulating and preventative properties. These herbs can be eaten in several ways, such as teas, tinctures, capsules, or by adding them to food.

Herbal antibiotics can be a natural method to support your health by preventing infections and boosting immunity. Following are some regularly used herbs, along with suggested dosage levels and techniques for preparation:

- **Echinacea**: Echinacea is well known for enhancing the immune system. It can be taken as a tincture, tea, or pill. For dose recommendations, refer to the product instructions. Echinacea is often taken for 7–10 days at a time, and there should be a 7–10-day gap before continuing.
- **Curcumin**: Curcumin, which is a compound present in turmeric, has anti-inflammatory and immune-boosting properties. Combine ground turmeric with warm milk or water to make a calming beverage. Increase the amount of turmeric you consume each day gradually as tolerated, starting with 1/4–1/2 teaspoon.
- **Andrographis**: An effective plant with immune-stimulating and anti-microbial effects. It is offered in pill and tincture form. Follow the dose guidelines mentioned or seek specific guidance from a healthcare provider.
- **Garlic**: Garlic possesses immune-boosting, antibacterial, and antiviral effects. It is better consumed uncooked since cooking could diminish its effectiveness. You can mince a garlic clove and add it to your dishes or blend it with honey. Although individual sensitivity levels can differ, a common dosage of 1-2 garlic cloves per day should be started with a small amount and increased gradually.
- **Ginger**: Ginger boosts the immune system and has antibacterial qualities. You can drink it as tea or include it in meals. Before straining and drinking the tea, several fresh ginger slices should be simmered in water for 10 to 15 minutes. You can drink up to four cups of ginger tea daily.
- **Honey:** Honey is said to be one of the oldest herbal antibiotics, being consumed since the ancient times. It boosts immunity and acts as a preventive measure to fight many bacteria. You can take a tablespoon of honey daily in the morning or you can a tablespoon of honey in a glass of warm water and consume it daily.

Despite the potential of herbal antibiotics, it's crucial to remember that everyone responds differently and that different dosages may be needed. Different dosages and formulations may be appropriate depending on the particular plant, a person's medical history, and other variables.

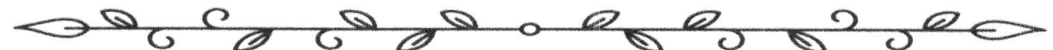

Before beginning any herbal regimen, seeking advice from a licensed healthcare provider or herbalist is essential, especially if you are on medication or have underlying medical conditions. Based on your unique requirements and circumstances, they can offer tailored advice just for you. Herbal antibiotics can enhance immune function and be a natural addition to a healthy lifestyle when used properly.

Summary

The usefulness and efficacy of employing herbal antibiotics for common ailments are examined in this chapter. For treating various medical issues and infections, herbal medicines present a safe and perhaps beneficial alternative to synthetic antibiotics. This chapter comprises the following aspects:

- Cuts, wounds, and skin infections can all be treated well with topical treatments of herbal antibiotics. Direct use of tea tree oil and garlic extracts, which have antibacterial and antiseptic qualities, can speed up healing and stop infection.
- Internal usage of herbal antibiotics is also possible for ailments like digestive problems and urinary tract infections (UTIs). Dandelion root, uva ursi, and cranberry are frequently utilized to maintain urinary health and prevent UTIs. Herbs like ginger, fennel, and peppermint can improve digestion, lessen inflammation, and combat gut bacterial overgrowth.
- Strong anti-microbial compounds in herbs like garlic, oregano, thyme, and tea tree oil can help fight bacterial, viral, and fungal diseases. These plants can be used in various ways, including oils, tinctures, extracts, topical applications, and oral formulations.
- Herbal antibiotics like thyme and eucalyptus can be inhaled for common conditions like respiratory infections or used for steam baths. This relieves symptoms, including coughs and sore throats, and helps to eliminate congestion. It also serves as a powerful antibacterial.
- The chapter also emphasizes the significance of seeing a specialist before taking herbal antibiotics for common conditions to ensure a proper diagnosis, suitable therapy, and personalized suggestions.

Incorporating herbal antibiotics into a holistic approach to wellness allows people to effectively treat common illnesses and can act as preventive measures against common ailments while reducing their risk of experiencing any adverse effects that may come with taking synthetic antibiotics. However, it's crucial to remember that for the best possible outcomes in terms of health, a precise diagnosis, expert counsel, and proper treatment are necessary.

Recipes for Health:
Making Your Own Herbal Antibiotics

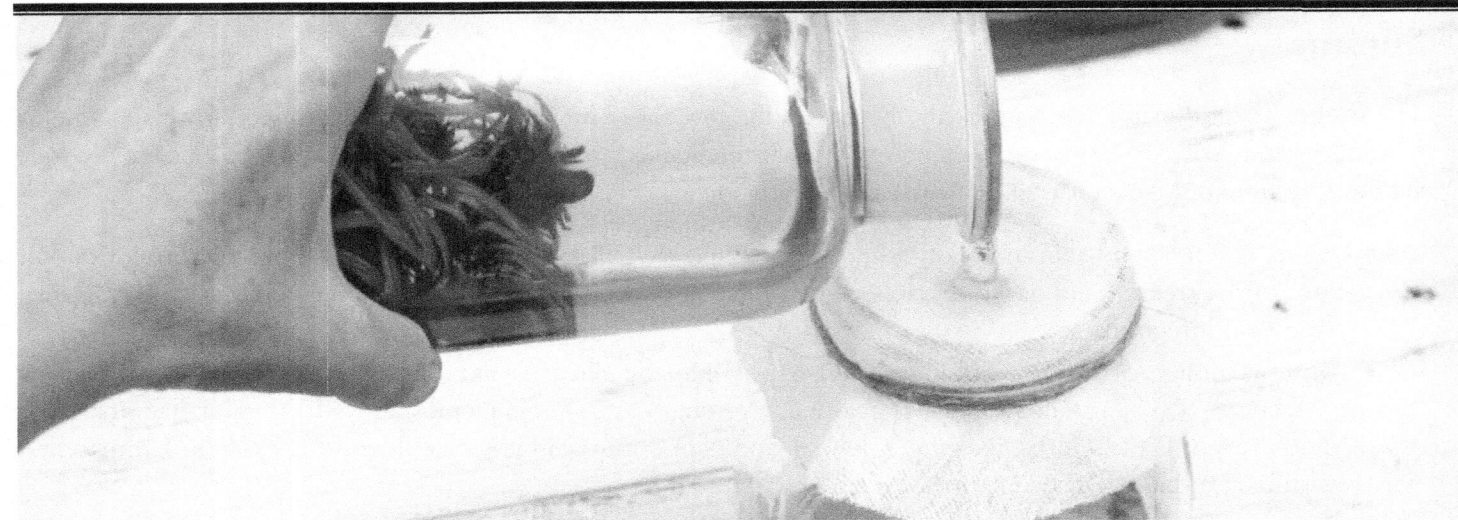

In every corner of the world, from bustling cities to quiet hamlets, people have relied upon the healing and nourishing powers of herbs. Herbal recipes, spanning millennia, have been handed down through generations, offering solutions for wellness, nutrition, and general well-being. These age-old formulations are nature's gift, tapping into the bounty of the Earth to support our body and mind.

The concept of herbal recipes revolves around harnessing the innate properties of herbs, spices, and other natural ingredients. Every herb, whether basil, thyme, or turmeric, carries its unique profile of nutrients, flavors, and medicinal properties. Combining these ingredients in specific ways can offer remedies for ailments, enhance flavor in our meals, or simply serve as a relaxation aid after a long day.

This section will delve deep into the world of herbal recipes. We'll uncover time-honored concoctions and modern interpretations, each with a detailed explanation. Whether you're looking for a calming herbal tea blend, a potent tincture for digestive health, or a fragrant herbal salve, we've got something for everyone. These recipes are about following instructions and understanding the "why" behind each ingredient's inclusion.

Creating your herbal recipes at home is a fulfilling journey. It's about being in sync with nature, understanding the rhythm of the seasons, and respecting the age-old wisdom accompanying each herb. It's also about customization, tailoring each recipe to your needs, preferences, and the specific challenges or desires you're addressing.

As we journey through these recipes, remember that while herbs offer immense benefits, it's essential to use them responsibly. Consider any allergies, consult with healthcare professionals if you're on medication or have specific health concerns, and always prioritize quality and purity when sourcing your ingredients.

Echinacea Tincture for Immune Support

Echinacea is widely regarded as one of nature's most potent immune boosters. Used traditionally by Native American tribes and later adopted and popularized in Western herbal medicine, this plant has been the subject of numerous scientific studies verifying its immune-modulating properties.

There are multiple ways to utilize the medicinal properties, but the most effective is making a tincture. Creating a tincture from echinacea allows easy ingestion and a longer shelf life, capturing the herb's beneficial properties in a concentrated form.

Ingredients:

- Fresh Echinacea root and aerial parts (flowers and leaves) - Approximately 2 cups
- High-proof alcohol (like vodka or brandy) - About 500 ml (2 cups)
- A glass jar with a tight-sealing lid (pint size or larger)
- Dark glass dropper bottles for storing the finished tincture

Step-by-Step Instructions:

- **Preparation of Herb:** Begin by carefully washing the fresh echinacea parts. Focus on washing and cleaning the plant and its parts from all the dirt. Chop them into smaller pieces to maximize the surface area.
- **Filling the Jar:** Place the chopped echinacea into your glass jar until it's about three-quarters full. Fresh echinacea will be used to maximize its benefits.
- **Adding the Alcohol:** Pour the high-proof alcohol over the echinacea in the jar, ensuring the plant material is fully submerged. If any parts stick out, they can mold or spoil the tincture. If needed, you can use more alcohol than the mentioned quantity; just make sure the echinacea is completely drowned in the liquid.
- **Sealing and Storing:** Place the lid on the jar and seal it tightly. Store the jar in a cool, dark place for 4-6 weeks. This is the extraction period, where the alcohol will pull the beneficial constituents out of the echinacea. Make sure not to move it around or keep it in direct sunlight, as this will destroy the herb's properties.
- **Daily Shake:** Remember to give your jar a good shake once a day during extraction.
- **Straining:** After 4-6 weeks, strain out the echinacea plant material using a fine mesh strainer or cheesecloth, capturing the liquid in a clean bowl or jug.
- **Bottling:** Transfer the strained liquid into dark glass dropper bottles using a funnel. These bottles protect the tincture from light, which can degrade its potency.
- **Labeling:** Always label your tinctures with the name and date of preparation. This ensures you know what's in the bottle and when it was made.

When to Use:
Take echinacea tincture when you feel you are about to have cold or flu to boost immune response. It can also be taken as a preventive measure during flu season or times of increased stress.

How to Use:
Standard Dose: A typical dose is 2-4 droppers full (about 2-4 ml) taken 2-3 times daily.

Duration: It's commonly recommended to take echinacea tincture for short periods (e.g., 2 weeks on, 1 week off) rather than continuously to maintain its effectiveness.

Like all herbal remedies, Echinacea tincture might not be suitable for everyone. Always consult a healthcare professional or herbalist before beginning any new herbal treatment, especially if you are pregnant, nursing, or on any medications.

Garlic Oil for Ear Infections

Garlic has been recognized since ancient times for its antimicrobial and anti-inflammatory properties. These characteristics make it a traditional remedy for various ailments, including ear infections.

Garlic oil is one of the oldest methods of medication extracted from garlic. It has useful remedies; the garlic oil helps most when warmed, it provides soothing relief from pain and helps combat the infection.

Ingredients:

- Fresh garlic cloves 3-4
- Olive oil or sweet almond oil 1/2 cup (approximately 120 ml)
- A small saucepan
- A fine mesh strainer or cheesecloth
- A glass jar or dropper bottle for storage

Step-by-Step Instructions:

- **Preparation of Garlic:** Start by peeling the garlic cloves, wash them and pat dry the cloves, and then finely mincing or crushing them. This action releases the allicin, a compound in garlic with potent antimicrobial properties.
- **Warming the Oil:** Pour the olive or sweet almond oil into a small saucepan. Warm the oil on low heat. You want it warm, not hot. The warmth in the oil will activate the oil nutrients, and infusing the oil with the benefits from the garlic cloves will become more fruitful.
- **Infusing the Oil:** Add the minced garlic to the warmed oil. Allow it to simmer on very low heat for about 20 minutes. Ensure the garlic doesn't fry or brown because high heat can destroy some beneficial properties.

- **Cooling and Straining:** After simmering, remove the saucepan and let the oil cool to room temperature. Once cooled, strain the garlic pieces using the strainer or cheesecloth, capturing the infused oil in a clean bowl or jug.
- **Storing:** Transfer the strained garlic oil into a clean glass jar or dropper bottle. Store in a cool, dark place, preferably in the refrigerator. Use within one month.

When to Use:

Use garlic oil at the first signs of an earache or ear infection. Remember, while garlic oil can relieve pain and may have antimicrobial properties, it's essential to consult with a healthcare provider to determine the cause of an earache and get appropriate treatment.

How to Use:

Warm the Oil: Warm the garlic oil before each use. You can do this by placing the dropper bottle or a small amount of the oil in a bowl of warm water for a few minutes. Test the temperature by placing a drop on the back of your hand to ensure it's not too hot.

Application: Using a dropper, put 2-3 drops of the warmed garlic oil into the affected ear while lying down with the affected ear facing upwards. Stay in this position for about 5-10 minutes, then place a cotton ball in the ear to prevent oil from dripping. Repeat 2-3 times a day as needed.

Caution: Do not use garlic oil if you suspect your eardrum is perforated or if there is any fluid draining from the ear. Always consult with a healthcare professional before using any home remedies. It is also better to use painkillers, other prescribed medicines, and garlic oil for faster relief.

Ginger Tea for Digestive Health

Ginger, a root hailed from Southeast Asia, has been embraced globally for its culinary and medicinal properties. Among its many benefits, ginger is particularly celebrated for promoting digestive health, alleviating nausea, and reducing bloating.

Numerous benefits are derived from a ginger root. One of the simplest and most effective ways to consume ginger for these benefits is tea. Drinking tea is an effective and quick way to remedy indigestion or bloating.

Ingredients:

- Fresh ginger root – 1-2 inches (2.5-5 cm)
- Water 2 cups or 475ml
- Optional: Honey or lemon slices for taste; it will also make the tea more effective with additional properties of lemon and/or honey.

Step-by-Step Instructions:

- **Preparing the Ginger:** First, thoroughly wash the ginger root to remove any dirt. Using a spoon or peeler, peel the skin off the ginger. Once peeled, thinly slice the ginger. The more surface area exposed, the stronger your tea will be. You must ensure that the peel is off as it does not contain any beneficial nutrients, but it may affect the taste of the tea and make it bitter.
- **Boiling:** Bring the 2 cups of water to a boil in a pot. Once boiling, add the ginger slices.
- **Simmering:** Reduce the heat to low and let the ginger simmer for 10-15 minutes. The longer you simmer, the stronger and more concentrated the tea will become.
- **Straining:** After simmering, remove the pot from the heat. Pour the tea into your cup using a filter, separating the liquid from the ginger slices.

- **Adding Flavors:** If desired, add honey or a slice of lemon to your tea for additional flavor and benefits. Honey can soothe the throat and provide sweetness, while lemon adds a refreshing taste and a dose of vitamin C.

When to Use:
Ginger tea is ideal for:

Post-Meals: If you've had a heavy meal and feel bloated. It would be best to have it something more complex for your stomach to digest after you have eaten, like some people can't digest whole corn.

Travelling: Especially if you are prone to motion sickness. If you are en route to a long journey, make some ginger tea and take it.

Morning Sickness: For pregnant women experiencing nausea (though it's crucial to consult with a healthcare provider first).

General Digestive Discomfort: Whenever you feel general unease in your stomach.

How to Use:
Sipping Slowly: Sip the tea slowly and let it work its magic to maximize its benefits. This is especially true if you're drinking it for nausea. Add a lemon wedge to make it taste better, and it will also benefit your nausea.

Frequency: You can drink ginger tea 2-3 times daily, depending on your need and tolerance. However, if you need it frequently, addressing the root cause of your digestive issues is essential.

While ginger tea is generally safe for most people, excessive consumption can lead to heartburn or stomach upset. It's always wise to start with a milder brew, especially if you're new to ginger tea. As with any remedy, consult a healthcare professional if you're pregnant, nursing, or on medication.

Goldenseal Salve for Skin Infection

Goldenseal, a native North American herb, is renowned for its potent antimicrobial and anti-inflammatory properties. Historically, Native American tribes used it for various ailments, and today, it remains a popular remedy, especially for skin issues.

Goldenseal is used to make a salve for skin issues. This salve, enriched with the essence of goldenseal, can be an effective balm for minor skin infections, cuts, and abrasions. It heals the area while keeping it hydrated and not making the area itchy.

Ingredients:

- Golden-seal root powder – 2 tablespoons
- Olive oil or sweet almond oil – 1 cup (approx. 240 ml)
- Beeswax – 2 oz (approximately 56 grams)
- Lavender essential oil (optional for scent and added antimicrobial properties) – 10-15 drops
- A double boiler or two pots
- Glass or metal tins or jars for storing the salve

Step-by-Step Instructions:

- **Infusing the Oil:** In the double boiler or using the two pots (one larger and filled with a bit of water, and a smaller one placed inside), warm the olive or sweet almond oil on low heat. Add the golden-seal root powder, stirring occasionally, and let it infuse for about 1-2 hours on very low heat. Ensure the oil does not overheat or boil. It is easier to make with golden-seal root powder as the infusion is efficient this way.
- **Straining the Oil:** Once infused, strain the oil through a fine mesh strainer or cheesecloth into a clean bowl or jar, removing all remnants of the golden-seal powder. the mesh cloth should be really fine to ensure that no powder gets mixed in the salve.
- **Melting the Beeswax:** Clean the double boiler or small pot and add the beeswax, allowing it to melt completely. Beeswax will give hydration and the required texture to the salve.
- **Combining Oil and Beeswax:** Once the beeswax is liquid, slowly pour in the infused oil, stirring constantly until the two are well combined. Do not stop stirring until both the liquids are unified.
- **Adding Essential Oil:** If you're using lavender essential oil or any other choice, now's the time to add it. Stir thoroughly. Make sure everything is mixed together well. Don't splash the mixture as it may still be hot to touch.
- **Setting the Salve:** While the mixture is still liquid, carefully pour it into your tins or jars, allowing it to cool and set at room temperature.
- **Storing:** Once solidified, cap your containers. Store them in a cool, dry place. Properly made and stored, the salve can last up to a year.

When to Use:
Use the golden-seal salve on minor skin infections, cuts, abrasions, or any skin irritation where antimicrobial action might be beneficial.

How to Use:
Application: Clean the affected area thoroughly. With clean fingers or a spatula, apply a small amount of the salve directly to the area. Cover with a bandage if needed.

Frequency: Depending on the severity of the issue, you can reapply the salve 2-3 times a day or as needed.

While goldenseal is generally considered safe for topical application, always do a patch test first to check for allergic reactions. Also, always consult a healthcare professional for severe or persistent skin issues or if you're unsure about using any new remedy.

Oregano Capsules for Respiratory Health

Oregano, a flavorful herb commonly used in culinary dishes, also boasts robust medicinal properties. Rich in Carvacrol and thymol, oregano has been suggested to promote respiratory health, provide antioxidant protection, and exert anti-inflammatory effects. Encapsulating oregano allows for easy and convenient consumption, especially for those who want to harness its health benefits.

Oregano capsules help make the respiratory system better. These capsules can be made at home by following the proper process described in this section.

Ingredients:

- Oregano leaf powder – 100 grams (ensure it is pure and free from additives or fillers)
- Empty gelatin or vegetarian capsules (Size "00") – approximately 150-200 capsules
- Capsule filling machine (optional but very useful)
- A clean tray or plate
- A small funnel or a piece of paper fashioned into a cone

Step-by-Step Instructions:

- **Preparing Workspace:** Ensure you have a clean, dry, and well-lit workspace. Lay out the tray or plate on which you'll work. If using a capsule filling machine, set it up according to the manufacturer's instructions. If doing it manually, it is better to wear gloves to ensure no bacteria is transferred.
- **Filling the Capsules:**
  - **Manual Method:** Open an empty capsule and hold the larger half. Using the funnel, pour the oregano leaf powder into the capsule, tapping gently to pack the powder down and fill the capsule as much as possible. Once filled, cap the capsule with the smaller half. As the capsule is size 00, it may be hard to work efficiently, and you will need practice to do it correctly.
  - **Capsule Machine:** If using a capsule filling machine, distribute the oregano powder over the machine, filling the capsule bases. Once all the capsules are filled, cap them according to the machine's instructions.
- **Storage:** Store the filled capsules in an airtight container away from direct sunlight, moisture, and heat. Keeping them in a cool, dark place will help preserve their potency. Ensure no moisture is added to the container as this will ruin the capsules.

When to Use:
Oregano capsules can be taken:

Cold and Flu Season: As a preventive measure during seasons when respiratory infections are rampant. It is necessary for those who suffer from chronic diseases like bronchitis or sinusitis.

Respiratory Discomfort: When experiencing symptoms like a mild cough or congestion. This may be due to the season or a viral going on.

How to Use:
Dosage: Typically, 1-2 capsules daily with a meal is recommended for adults. However, this can vary based on the individual and the concentration of the oregano powder.

Duration: While oregano can be taken as a daily supplement, it's always best to take breaks. For example, one might take it for 2-3 weeks, followed by a week off.

Caution: It's crucial to consult with a healthcare provider before starting any new supplement, including oregano capsules, especially for pregnant or nursing women, children, or those on medication. Some individuals might experience digestive upset or allergic reactions from oregano. Always start with a lower dose to assess tolerance. Discontinue usage if any discomfort is caused after 2-3 doses.

Thyme Syrup for Cough

Thyme, a fragrant herb with small, delicate leaves, has been cherished for ages not just for its culinary uses but also for its therapeutic benefits. Rich in thymol and other bio-active compounds, thyme has demonstrated antimicrobial and anti-inflammatory properties, making it an excellent remedy for coughs and respiratory ailments.

Thyme syrup for cough is proven to ease cough and discomfort in the throat. This syrup harnesses the goodness of thyme in a palatable form. It is safe to be used for any age group as it is chemical-free.

Ingredients:

- Fresh thyme leaves – 1 cup (packed) or Dried thyme – 1/2 cup
- Raw honey – 1 cup (approx. 240 ml)
- Filtered water – 2 cups (approx. 475 ml)
- Optional: Juice of 1 lemon for added flavor and vitamin C

Step-by-Step Instructions:

- **Preparing Thyme Infusion:** In a saucepan, bring the filtered water to a boil. Once boiling, reduce the heat and add the thyme leaves (either fresh or dried). Let it simmer for about 10-15 minutes. The flame should be low so that the infusion process is optimum.
- **Straining the Infusion:** After simmering, remove the saucepan from heat. Strain the liquid to remove the thyme leaves, pouring the infusion into a bowl or jug. Allow it to cool slightly, but not entirely. It should be warm enough to dissolve the honey but not so hot as to destroy its beneficial enzymes. Scalding hot water will kill all the beneficial elements of the water, so make sure it is warm before you add the honey to the filtered and infused water.
- **Adding Honey:** Pour honey into the warm thyme infusion, stirring constantly to ensure it dissolves completely. If you're using lemon juice, add it now. Keep stirring to unify the ingredients so that the thyme infusion in the water gets mixed with honey and lemon (if added).
- **Bottling the Syrup:** Once the honey is dissolved, pour the syrup into a sterilized glass bottle or jar. Seal it tightly. The bottle should be airtight.
- **Storage:** Store the thyme syrup in the refrigerator. It should remain potent for 4-6 weeks. Use a clean spoon to take the syrup each time; do not use a dirty or used and unwashed spoon so that no unnecessary bacteria enter your body.

When to Use:
Thyme syrup can be taken

At the Onset of a Cough or Cold: To alleviate symptoms and speed up recovery.

Chronic Respiratory Conditions: A natural supplement to soothe the throat and reduce coughing episodes.

How to Use:

Dosage for Adults: 1-2 tablespoons every 3-4 hours or as needed.

Dosage for Children (over one-year-old): 1-2 teaspoons every 3-4 hours or as needed. Do not give honey-based syrups to infants under 12 months due to the risk of botulism.

Serving Suggestions: The syrup can be taken independently or mix it into a warm cup of tea or water.

Ask a healthcare provider before starting any herbal remedy, especially if pregnant, nursing, giving to children, or taking medication. Allergies to thyme are uncommon but not unheard of, so it's good to be cautious.

Turmeric Paste for Inflammation

Turmeric, a golden-hued root native to South Asia, has been utilized for millennia in traditional Ayurveda and Chinese medicine. Curcumin, the active compound in turmeric, is praised for its potent anti-inflammatory and antioxidant benefits.

Turmeric can be used in multiple forms, a paste can be applied topically for skin issues or pains, as well as taken orally for inflammation and other gut-related issues. This turmeric paste, sometimes known as "Golden Paste," concentrates the power of turmeric in a palatable, versatile form.

Ingredients:

- Turmeric powder – 1/2 cup (approximately 60 grams)
- Filtered water – 1 cup (approximately 240 ml)
- Black pepper, freshly ground – 1 1/2 teaspoons (black pepper enhances the absorption of curcumin in the body)
- Coconut oil or extra virgin olive oil – 1/4 cup (approximately 60 ml)

Step-by-Step Instructions:

- **Preparing the Turmeric Base:** In a saucepan, combine the turmeric powder with filtered water. Mix well to form a smooth paste. There should be no lumps and the paste should not stick to the pan.
- **Cooking the Paste:** Place the saucepan on medium heat. Stir continuously to prevent the paste from sticking or forming lumps. As the mixture heats, it will start to thicken. This process may take a few moments as the water dries up and the turmeric starts dissolving.
- **Adding Oil and Pepper:** Once the paste reaches a thick consistency (similar to a soft dough), reduce the heat and stir in the freshly ground black pepper and coconut or olive oil.

Mix well to ensure even distribution. The oil will give it a shine and nice consistency, while pepper will give flavor to it. Black pepper also has healing properties but cannot be consumed in higher quantities.

- **Cooling and Storing:** Remove the paste from heat and allow it to cool down. Once cooled, transfer the turmeric paste into a clean glass jar with a tight-fitting lid. Store in the refrigerator for up to 2-3 weeks.

When to Use:
Turmeric paste can be used:

Daily Wellness Routine: As a preventive measure to keep inflammation at bay and promote overall health.

Inflammatory Conditions: To alleviate symptoms of conditions such as arthritis, muscle pain, or any inflammation-related discomfort.

How to Use:
Dosage for Adults: Start with 1/4 teaspoon daily, gradually increasing to 1-2 teaspoons per day, as your body gets accustomed to it. If you feel like you are not liking the flavor you can add a few drops of honey to it or take the paste with some other ingredient like milk or warm water.

Serving Suggestions: You can mix the paste into warm milk or tea, often referred to as "Golden Milk." Additionally, it can be incorporated into smoothies, soups, or any dish that complements its flavor. Some even consume it directly. Directly, it may taste unlikeable, but it is more potent if taken on its own.

Consult a healthcare provider before starting any new supplement or remedy, especially if pregnant, nursing, or on medication. Turmeric is generally safe, but in large doses or for specific individuals, it may cause stomach upset or interfere with certain medications. Always do a patch test if applying topically to ensure there are no allergic reactions.

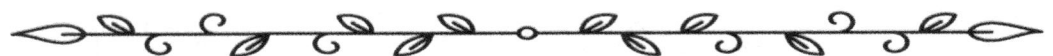

More Natural Remedies

In addition to the natural remedies already mentioned, you can discover a comprehensive selection tailored for various ailments, ranging from sore throats and bronchitis to menstrual cramps and headaches. To access this information, you may either visit the provided link or scan the QR code.

https://www.wiseapublishing.com/herbalAB/bonus/

Summary

In our comprehensive exploration of herbal remedies, we delved deep into the profiles and medicinal applications of several herbs known for their therapeutic properties:

- **Echinacea:** Esteemed for its immune-boosting abilities, we outlined the preparation of an echinacea tincture. This tincture capitalizes on echinacea attributes to fortify the immune system, making it a potential ally during cold and flu seasons. It can be taken by adults, but the quantity must be limited.
- **Garlic:** A household name, garlic's prowess goes beyond the culinary domain. We discussed the formulation of garlic oil tailored for ear infections, taking advantage of its natural antimicrobial properties. One should keep the ear facing upward for at least 5 minus after putting the oil in.
- **Ginger:** Known for its zesty flavor and health-promoting qualities, ginger was presented as tea. This ginger tea can be a soothing remedy, particularly beneficial for digestive health.
- **Goldenseal:** This herb's potential in combating skin infections was captured in the recipe for goldenseal salve. A natural ointment that could be a boon for minor cuts, scrapes, or skin irritations.
- **Oregano:** While it's a staple in Mediterranean cuisine, oregano's therapeutic potential is encapsulated, quite literally, in our discussion on oregano capsules. These capsules, packed with compounds beneficial for respiratory health, are ideal during respiratory distress or as a preventive measure. Do not use the capsules as a supplement or for a longer period, discontinue use after 2 weeks maximum.
- **Thyme:** We ventured into preparing a thyme syrup tailored for cough relief. Harnessing thyme's natural anti-tussive properties, this syrup can be a gentle remedy for persistent coughs or respiratory discomfort.
- **Turmeric:** Celebrated for its anti-inflammatory properties, we crafted a recipe for turmeric paste, sometimes called "Golden Paste." This potent concoction can be a daily supplement for those looking to mitigate inflammation or simply for overall wellness.

Each of these herbal preparations was accompanied by detailed instructions, dosages, and applications, providing a holistic guide for anyone interested in herbal remedies. Whether you're a seasoned herbalist or a curious novice, these insights offer a window into the vast world of plant-based healing.

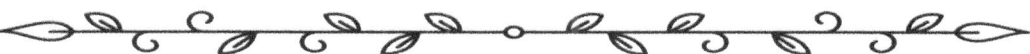

The Future of Herbal Antibiotics: Trends and Predictions

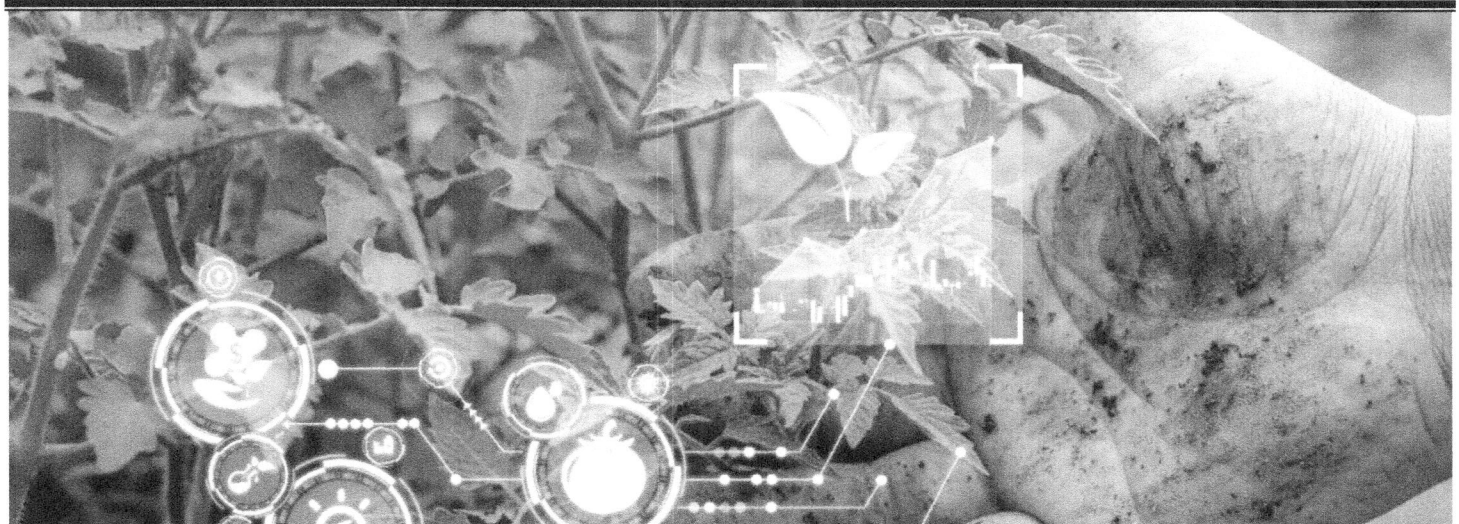

Herbal antibiotics have been nature's ancient gift, standing at the crossroads where tradition meets modern science. As we increasingly navigate a world grappling with antibiotic resistance and the pursuit of holistic health, herbal antibiotics' future appears promising and pivotal.

The medicines sourced through herbs are easier to get and can have multiple benefits on the health. Let's explore this intriguing confluence.

Current Trends in Herbal Antibiotics

Herbal medicine has been in use for most of human history. Herbs have been used to make multiple treatments that can be administered topically and orally. Herbal antibiotics have been in a trial period for the longest time, and still, much research is being done on different medicines. There are a few reasons for the popularity of herbal medicine that is growing again.

- **Rising Popularity:** Many are seeking alternatives, with antibiotic resistance becoming a global health threat. Herbal antibiotics are gaining traction as potential alternatives or supplements to pharmaceutical antibiotics. Plants like garlic, echinacea, and goldenseal, once household remedies, are now being revisited with renewed interest.
- **Trends in Use:** The modern user is keen on preventive health. Prophylactic usage of herbal antibiotics, aimed at bolstering the immune system rather than treating a full-blown infection, is a trending practice.

Studies of Herbal Antibiotics:

- **Scientific Validation:** Modern science is increasingly investigating the efficacy of herbal antibiotics. Rigorous studies, clinical trials, and meta-analyses are underway to understand the exact mechanisms, potential drug-herb interactions, and ideal dosages.
- **Integrated Pharmaco-botany:** Modern labs are employing techniques like gas chromatography and mass spectrometry to isolate and study the active compounds in herbs. This integrated approach, blending botany with pharmacology, is producing groundbreaking insights.

Increased Interest in Natural Health Solutions:

- **Return to Roots:** A sizeable portion of the global population actively seeks organic, natural remedies. This shift in preference stems from concerns about synthetic drug side effects, a desire for sustainable health solutions, and a growing trust in nature-derived therapies.
- **Global Fusion:** Western consumers are embracing practices from Ayurveda, Traditional Chinese Medicine, and African Traditional Healing, expanding the repertoires of known herbal antibiotics and introducing a plethora of new plant-based treatments.

Integration of Traditional and Modern Science:

- **Collaborative Approach:** Traditional knowledge holders and modern scientists collaborate, ensuring that the ancient wisdom of herbal antibiotics is translated effectively and safely for contemporary use.
- **Technological Aids:** Advanced technologies like AI and machine learning are being employed to predict potential uses of herbs, analyze vast traditional texts, and optimize extraction processes for maximum potency.

In essence, the future of herbal antibiotics is shimmering with potential. As humanity progresses, it seems we are also taking a moment to look back, reconnect with the Earth, and harness the healing powers that nature has generously provided. Traditional wisdom and modern science walk hand in hand in this journey, leading us toward a brighter, healthier tomorrow.

Emerging Research in Herbal Antibiotics

The landscape of health and wellness is witnessing a renewed interest in plant-derived compounds, especially as the spectre of antibiotic resistance looms. Recent research in herbal antibiotics is groundbreaking, taking a holistic approach while building upon age-old knowledge.

Herbal or plant-based medicine is promising and provides solutions to common illnesses. Another big benefit of plant-based medicine is the side effects are low and non-life threatening, which can be contrary to synthetic medicines. Let's delve deeper into these promising investigations.

Recent Findings in Herbal Antibiotics:

- **Multi-drug Resistant Bacteria and Phyto-compounds:** Some recent studies have shown that certain plant compounds are effective against multi-drug resistant strains of bacteria. For instance, research on compounds like berberine (found in golden-seal) and allicin (from garlic) have shown promise against such hard-to-treat strains. The complex compound aims for more than one type of bacteria or treats more than one organ at once. This benefit outweighs the minor side effects.
- **Synergy with Conventional Antibiotics:** Herbal compounds, in some cases, have been found to enhance the efficacy of conventional antibiotics. This synergistic effect can lead to reduced dosages and fewer side effects. A study published in the journal "PLOS ONE" suggested that certain herbal compounds disrupt bacterial cell walls when used with traditional antibiotics, making the bacteria more susceptible. As the saying goes, 'two is better than one', similar is the case with medicine. To maximize the chances of treating a chronic or fatal illness, a combination of herbal with synthetic medicine may provide better solutions.
- **Herbal Biofilms:** A groundbreaking area of research revolves around bacterial biofilms, which are protective layers that bacteria form to shield themselves from antibiotics. Some herbs, like oregano and thyme, have demonstrated the potential to disrupt these biofilms, paving the way for more effective treatment. The penetration in the bacteria with the help of plant-based medicine helps counter the disease on a deeper level instead of just suppressing the bacteria.

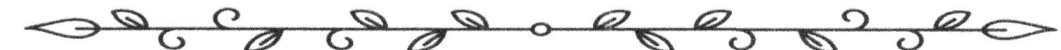

Potential Implications of These Findings:

- **Natural Solutions to Antibiotic Resistance:** With antibiotic resistance being one of our most pressing health challenges, these findings indicate that herbal antibiotics might be part of the solution. They offer pathways to develop newer effective treatments that are less likely to induce resistance. Antibiotic resistance may not be treatable with other harsh antibiotics. Still, with herbal options, there may be a way to treat or reverse the resistance.

- **Pharmaceutical Integration:** These discoveries may lead to the integration of herbal compounds into mainstream pharmaceuticals. Instead of viewing herbal and conventional treatments as separate entities, future medications might beautifully blend the two, offering the best of both worlds. The research and experimentation may still take time, but the future holds better medication through a synergy of both medicines.

- **Holistic Approaches to Health:** The research underscore the importance of a holistic approach to health. Instead of targeting a single aspect of the bacterium, herbal antibiotics often work on multiple fronts – from disrupting biofilms to enhancing the body's immune responses. Herbal antibiotics reach more than one area in the body that may be affected by the bacteria, unlike synthetic medicine, which focuses on one issue at a time. Herbal medicine treats the illness from the root instead of just brushing it under the carpet.

- **Personalized Medicine:** With the increased understanding of herbal antibiotics, we're inching closer to tailored treatments. As genetic profiling and personalized medicine advance, individuals might receive treatments based on their unique genetic makeup, optimizing efficacy and reducing side effects. It is a beneficial solution for fatal or complex diseases or multiple diseases endured by a single person. A customized medicine or plan or medicines will help the doctors with treating the patient efficiently.

- **Conservation and Sustainability:** As the importance of these plants becomes more recognized, there will be an impetus towards their conservation and sustainable cultivation. Ensuring a continuous supply while preserving biodiversity will be pivotal. The plants need a certain type of atmosphere (each plant has its own specific requirements), this is a challenge to do if the medication is to be produced on a large scale. Facilities with proper care and techniques to let the plans thrive and reach the optimum stage will have to be made.

In summary, the horizon of herbal antibiotic research is vast and expanding. As modern science deepens its understanding of these ancient remedies, we stand at the cusp of a revolution that respects nature, integrates diverse knowledge systems, and seeks to provide the most holistic care for all.

Predictions for Future Herbal Antibiotics

Gazing into the crystal ball of herbal antibiotics, the interplay of age-old wisdom, emerging research, and contemporary health challenges creates a complex but promising panorama. The medicine industry is set toward advancement by stepping ahead in research and discovering alternatives to pharmaceutical antibiotics using herbal medicine.

The field is ever evolving, and the predictions are also changing with time. Some decades ago, no one was ready to return to herbal medicines as traditional or synthetic medicine evolved. But now, people are more interested in the natural way of healing their bodies without exposing themselves to fatal side effects. Based on current trends and research breakthroughs, here are some informed predictions about the trajectory of herbal antibiotics.

1. Mainstream Acceptance and Integration:

- **Integrated Medicine:** Traditional and modern medical practices will become more intertwined. Expect more doctors and healthcare providers to recommend herbal antibiotics alongside or in place of pharmaceutical

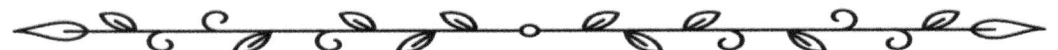

antibiotics, especially for mild infections or prophylactic use. This benefits the human body and the environment, as herbal medicines are cost-effective and create almost no un-recyclable waste.

- **Pharmaceutical Adaptations:** Major pharmaceutical companies will likely invest in research and development of hybrid drugs, combining synthetic compounds with herbal extracts, aiming to leverage the synergistic effects and improve efficacy. The steps of adaptation will be a game-changer as more people will get treatment without taking strong synthetic chemicals.

2. Personalized Herbal Treatments:

- **Genomics Medicine:** As the field of genomics expands, we may see individualized herbal treatments tailored to patients' genetic profiles. This could maximize efficacy while minimizing adverse reactions. This was also a tradition in the old times; herbal medicines like teas or syrups were made keeping in mind the person's preference; taste and sweetness or bitterness were adjusted using other available in-kitchen ingredients.
- **AI & Big Data:** With advancements in artificial intelligence, vast data from traditional medicine can be analyzed in-depth. AI can help predict which herbal compounds can be effective against specific pathogens or conditions, leading to targeted treatments. The information from AI can be a big step forward.

3. Sustainable Sourcing and Conservation:

- **Eco-friendly Cultivation:** With the rising demand for medicinal plants, sustainable farming practices will become paramount. This will ensure a steady supply without depleting or endangering wild populations.
- **Bio-piracy Concerns:** As the value of these herbs becomes widely recognized, there will be heightened discussions around intellectual property rights, especially concerning indigenous knowledge and the potential exploitation of native resources. The origination of the herbs will be given importance, and more research will be done to maximize the benefits.

4. Comprehensive Studies and Quality Control:

- **Standardization:** With herbal antibiotics gaining prominence, there will be a push for standardization. This means producing herbal products with consistent quality, potency, and safety. It will be a huge step as developed and first-world countries aim to provide healthcare of the same quality for everyone.
- **In-depth Research:** Beyond efficacy, research will delve deeper into understanding these herbs' mechanisms, possibly leading to new therapeutic pathways or techniques.

5. Holistic Health Movement:

- **Lifestyle Medicine:** The broader movement towards holistic health will see individuals integrating herbal antibiotics as remedies and as part of daily routines to maintain wellness. Herbal supplements are a part of daily routine in some South Asian countries, but it will be more common.
- **Educational Initiatives:** As the populace becomes more health-conscious, there'll be increased demand for educational resources about herbal antibiotics — their benefits, risks, and best practices. Understanding the herbs, their potency, and the optimum health benefits will be unveiled with time.

6. Policy Changes and Regulation:

- **Governmental Support:** We might witness more governmental agencies promoting research into herbal antibiotics, especially as antibiotic resistance escalates. Herbal antibiotics and medicines are evolving to present beneficial alternatives to harsh antibiotics; it is a win-win situation.

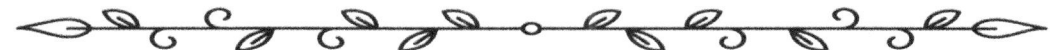

- **Stricter Regulations:** As the market for herbal antibiotics expands, regulations will tighten to ensure consumer safety and product efficacy. The manufacturing will be large-scale, similar to the traditional pharmaceutical medicines, and regulations will be set keeping in mind the safety rules for everyone's health.

In essence, the future of herbal antibiotics is dynamic and brimming with possibilities. As global challenges like antibiotic resistance intensify and our understanding of nature's pharmacy deepens, herbal antibiotics are poised to play an even more crucial role in our collective health and well-being.

Role of Herbal Antibiotics in Global Health

The contemporary global health landscape is fraught with challenges — from antibiotic resistance to inequalities in healthcare access. Herbal antibiotics, with their ancient roots and emerging scientific validation, can be critical in reshaping this landscape. Let's unpack the significance of herbal antibiotics in addressing global health concerns.

1. Tackling Antibiotic Resistance:

- **Natural Alternatives:** As many bacterial strains evolve to resist synthetic antibiotics, herbal antibiotics offer alternative treatment pathways. These natural compounds might act on bacteria differently, reducing the chance of resistance development. Nature-derived medicine's complexity will strengthen the body and combat any other dangerous bacteria before it can spread.
- **Synergy with Synthetic Antibiotics:** Some herbal antibiotics have shown promise in enhancing the efficacy of conventional drugs, potentially reducing the required dose and decreasing the likelihood of resistance emergence. The herbal medicines are known to work slowly but efficiently. A person can treat most minor illnesses like a cold, flu, or fever just by consuming different types of teas, and this means that the immunity is strengthened to fight the bacteria on its own without introducing it to any foreign chemicals.

2. Bridging the Healthcare Access Gap:

- **Cost-Effective Treatment:** Many herbal remedies can be sourced locally and produced at a fraction of the cost of synthetic drugs, making them accessible to under-served populations. Most developing countries rely on poor healthcare systems as healthcare costs are very high. Herbal alternatives will be able to provide equal healthcare to everyone.
- **Local Cultivation:** Communities can be trained to cultivate and process their medicinal plants, ensuring a steady supply and generating local income. This may depend on the climate and seasons experienced by the local area, but greenhouses and shaded or artificial lighting can also solve this issue.
- **Traditional Knowledge Utilization:** Leveraging indigenous medical knowledge can help customize treatments according to local needs and cultural preferences.

3. Promoting Preventive Health:

- **Holistic Well-being:** Beyond their antibiotic properties, many medicinal herbs have multifaceted health benefits, promoting overall wellness and disease prevention. Many herbal medicines do not have age restrictions; kids can also have the cough syrup dosage without the fear of severe side effects.
- **Enhancing Immunity:** Some herbal antibiotics, like echinacea and garlic, combat pathogens and bolster the body's natural defenses.

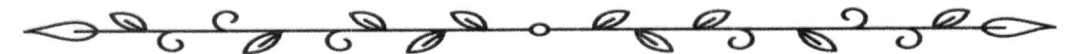

4. Reducing Dependency on the Pharmaceutical Supply Chain:

- **Local Solutions to Local Problems:** Herbal antibiotics can be cultivated and processed locally, reducing dependency on global pharmaceutical supply chains, which can be vulnerable to disruptions.
- **Decentralized Healthcare:** Herbal treatments promote a decentralized approach, enabling communities to address specific health issues autonomously, without waiting for external aid or supplies.

5. Environmental and Biodiversity Benefits:

- **Sustainable Farming:** Encouraging the cultivation of medicinal plants can promote biodiversity and sustainable farming practices. The plantation will benefit the local area's weather and air quality positively.
- **Conservation Efforts:** Recognizing the medicinal value of certain plants can spur conservation efforts, ensuring the preservation of valuable ecosystems.

6. Cultural and Socio-economic Aspects:

- **Preserving Heritage:** Emphasizing the importance of herbal medicine can help preserve cultural heritage and traditional medical practices.
- **Empowerment:** Equipping communities with the knowledge and means to harness their local flora for health can lead to empowerment and self-reliance.

The role of herbal antibiotics in global health is multifaceted and profound. As we grapple with modern health challenges, these ancient remedies offer hope in battling diseases and fostering a more inclusive, sustainable, and resilient healthcare paradigm.

Preparing for the Future: How to Stay Informed

The world of herbal antibiotics is vast and continually evolving. As the importance of these natural remedies becomes increasingly apparent, individuals must stay updated on the latest findings, practices, and insights. Here are some strategies and resources to ensure you remain well-informed about developments in herbal antibiotics.

1. Academic Journals and Publications:

- **Stay Subscribed:** Regularly check reputable journals related to herbal medicine, pharmacology, and ethnobotany. Journals such as Phytomedicine, Journal of Ethnopharmacology, and Journal of Herbal Medicine offer peer-reviewed research.
- **Access Databases:** Utilize academic databases like PubMed, ScienceDirect, and Google Scholar. These platforms collate various research articles, reviews, and case studies related to herbal medicine.

2. Join Professional Organizations:

- **Network and Learn:** Bodies like the American Herbalists Guild or the National Institute of Medical Herbalists often host seminars, workshops, and conferences. These events can be a goldmine of new information and networking opportunities.
- **Access Exclusive Resources:** Membership in such organizations might grant you access to exclusive publications, research databases, and expert consultations.

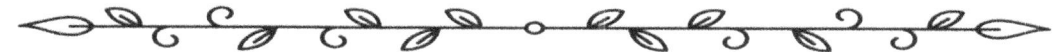

3. Online Courses and Workshops:

- **Stay Educated:** Websites like Coursera, Udemy, and edX often host courses on herbal medicine, ranging from beginner to advanced levels.
- **Interactive Learning:** Workshops, either virtual or in-person, can offer hands-on experiences, like making herbal concoctions or identifying medicinal plants.

4. Engage with Communities:

- **Online Forums and Groups:** Platforms like Reddit and Facebook have numerous groups dedicated to herbal medicine where members share articles, and personal experiences and answer queries.
- **Local Herbalist Circles:** Many regions have local herbalist groups that organize meetings, plant walks, and other informative events.

5. Books and Periodicals:

- **Stay Updated with Publications:** New books on herbal medicine are published frequently. Keep an eye out for works by renowned herbalists or researchers. Periodicals or magazines dedicated to herbal medicine can also be a treasure trove of information.

6. Collaborate with Universities or Research Institutions:

- **Research Partnerships:** If you're sincerely interested or involved in the field, consider collaborating with universities or institutions with ethnobotany or herbal medicine departments. Such partnerships can offer in-depth insights and early access to cutting-edge findings.

7. Monitor News Outlets:

- **Relevant News Sections:** Mainstream news outlets sometimes cover significant breakthroughs in herbal medicine, especially concerning public health.
- **Specialized Blogs and Websites:** Numerous websites and blogs are dedicated to herbal medicine. Subscribing to them can keep you updated with the latest trends and findings.

In essence, staying informed in the dynamic realm of herbal antibiotics requires a multi-pronged approach. By leveraging the resources above and fostering a genuine curiosity about the field, you can remain at the forefront of herbal antibiotic knowledge and practice.

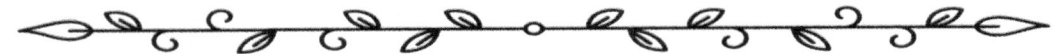

Summary

Throughout our exploration of herbal antibiotics, we've traversed a range of topics, from individual herb profiles and their diverse applications to emerging research that underscores their potential. The takeaway is clear: the significance of herbal antibiotics in the contemporary health scene is undeniable and poised to grow even further.

While modern medicine has undoubtedly transformed healthcare, bringing myriad innovations and solutions, the rise of issues like antibiotic resistance has necessitated a pivot. Herbal antibiotics have emerged as promising allies in this challenging landscape with their rich history and newfound validations.

- Emerging research has brought exciting revelations to the fore. Modern science is continually unearthing new dimensions of these herbs, corroborating ancient wisdom with empirical evidence. This synergy between the old and the new holds immense promise as it bridges traditional practices with contemporary needs.
- Predictions based on current trends suggest that the reliance on and interest in herbal antibiotics will only amplify. Their potential role in global health is especially significant, offering solutions to challenges like antibiotic resistance and healthcare disparities.
- Moreover, staying informed, as we've highlighted, is crucial. The world of herbal antibiotics is dynamic, with new findings and insights emerging regularly. Harnessing this potential requires proactive learning and a commitment to understanding the intricacies of the field.

The convergence of tradition and modern science in herbal antibiotics represents a beacon of hope. As we navigate the complexities of modern health challenges, these natural remedies stand as a testament to the enduring power of nature and its unparalleled potential to shape the future of health and medicine.

Conclusion:
Your Journey Towards Natural Health

Navigating the vast landscape of health and wellness, you've now embarked on a journey rooted in ancient wisdom and modern understanding: the world of herbal antibiotics. This journey is not just a personal exploration but a step towards a more sustainable and holistic approach to global health.

Herbal antibiotics have been the bedrock of traditional healing systems across cultures and epochs. Their value arises not just from treating symptoms, as many modern medicines do, but by often addressing the root cause of ailments, promoting overall well-being, and enhancing body resilience.

Comparatively, while traditional antibiotics have been groundbreaking in battling numerous diseases and saving countless lives, they come with their own set of challenges. Over-reliance on them has led to antibiotic resistance, a burgeoning global health crisis. The side effects and imbalances caused by these synthetic drugs are also of concern. In contrast, herbal antibiotics, when used correctly, tend to work in harmony with the body, fortifying it rather than creating imbalances.

As you shift towards herbal antibiotics, you'll discover many benefits:

- **Holistic Healing:** Herbal remedies often focus on total body wellness, aiding not just the ailment in question but contributing to overall health.
- **Reduced Side Effects:** Herbal antibiotics, being natural, usually have fewer side effects when compared to synthetic drugs.
- **Sustainability:** Herbal remedies can be more sustainable, with a reduced carbon footprint, especially if sourced locally or grown at home.
- **Empowerment:** Knowledge of herbal remedies empowers individuals to take charge of their health, understanding what they consume and its implications.

Adapting to herbal antibiotics necessitates a commitment to understanding, patience, and often a paradigm shifts in how one perceives health. It's about reconnecting with nature, understanding its rhythms, and recognizing the symbiotic relationship humans share with the natural world.

However, one must approach this transition with prudence. While herbal antibiotics offer many benefits, they are not a replacement for all modern medicines. It's essential to consult with healthcare professionals, especially when dealing with severe ailments or when merging herbal remedies with other medications.

In the grand tapestry of global health, the resurgence of interest in herbal antibiotics is a glimmer of hope. As individuals and communities gravitate towards these natural remedies, there's potential for a health revolution - one that's grounded in nature, respects the body's innate healing capacities, and addresses the emerging challenges of our times.

Your journey towards natural health using herbal antibiotics is not just a personal health choice. It's a step towards a future where health is holistic, sustainable, and harmonious with the natural world.

Made in the USA
Las Vegas, NV
09 February 2025